Web Health
Information Resources

Web Health Information Resources

For Consumers, Healthcare Providers, Patients and Physicians

Second Edition

Eugene A. DeFelice, M.D.

iUniverse, Inc.

New York   Lincoln   Shanghai

Web Health Information Resources
For Consumers, Healthcare Providers, Patients and Physicians

iUniverse, Inc.

For information address:
iUniverse, Inc.
2021 Pine Lake Road, Suite 100
Lincoln, NE 68512
www.iuniverse.com

ISBN: 0-595-32628-5

Printed in the United States of America

Dedication

This book is dedicated to Ms. Maryanne Harvey, M.S. and Mr. Benjamin (Ben) DeFelice.

Maryanne has devoted her professional career to the betterment of the health and welfare of others as a member of the New York State Department of Health, which she now serves as a consultant. Without Maryanne's able professional advice and assistance, publication of this book would not have been possible.

Ben, my brother, world traveler, raconteur extraordinaire, friend and helping hand to many throughout his life, a "man for all seasons", served as my Literary Agent regarding publication of this book.

Contents

Acknowledgements

The author acknowledges that the Web Health Resources/Websites in the Author's List, and additional ones cited in the text, provided the information presented in this book and are hereby credited accordingly.

Special thanks also go to the J. Spencer and Patricia Standish Library of Siena College, in Loudonville, New York and Niagara University, Niagara Falls, New York for the use of their library/computer facilities and assistance provided by their Reference Librarians in researching the subject matter for this book.

Preface

Most individuals do not live a healthy lifestyle or devote sufficient attention to their health and wellness. If you are one of those who do not, bear in mind that:

You may squander health in search of wealth
Work and toil and save
Then squander wealth in search of health
Only to find an early grave.

Anonymous.

A healthy lifestyle is essential for good health and longevity. An unhealthy one leads to chronic diseases and a shortened lifespan. Chronic disorders such as heart disease, cancer, and diabetes are among the leading causes of disability and premature death in the United States. In fact, these diseases account for around 7 out of every 10 deaths and affect the quality of life of the majority of adult Americans. Chronic diseases are not only among the most common but also among the most preventable. Adopting a healthy lifestyle, eating a sensible and nutritious diet, becoming physically active and avoiding tobacco and excessive alcohol use not only may prevent but also may control the devastating effects of chronic diseases, once present. This book provides you with a number of Key Web Health Resources to help you achieve these goals. Bear in mind that stress control, mindfulness and spirituality are also considered to be important aspects of a healthy lifestyle and a number of key Web Health Resources are made available on these subjects as well.

It now is estimated that over 200-300 million adults in the Western World use the Web to obtain health and wellness information, and over 75% find such useful. By using the Web for health and wellness information, you also may be rewarded accordingly.

This book provides only those Web Resources and corresponding Websites that are considered to be reasonably trustworthy and provide current, comprehensive, reliable and useful information on a wide variety of health and wellness subjects. However, in order to obtain the "best available information", you need to ask the "right questions" and seek appropriate answers. In this regard, it has been said:

> I keep six honest serving men
> They taught me all I knew
> Their names are What and Why and When
> And How and Where and Who.
>
> *Rudyard Kipling*

Asking the "right questions" and obtaining the "best available information" enables you to become knowledgeable and take charge, control, and responsibility regarding your health and wellness. With the "best information" in hand, you can make informed decisions with your healthcare provider/physician, and live a healthier, happier, longer, and more productive/enjoyable life.

However, in obtaining such information, remember:

> Read not to contradict and confute,
> nor to believe and take for granted,
> nor to talk and discourse, but to weigh and consider.
>
> *Francis Bacon*

> Every truth passes through three stages before
> it is recognized. In the first, it is ridiculed.
> In the second, it is opposed. In the third, it is
> regarded as self-evident.
>
> *Schopenhauer*

In order to be a better patient, you need to become fully involved in your healthcare and wellness, and seek out all pertinent information from the Web in order to do so. However, in so doing, always take care to be reasonably certain that the information you obtain/use comes from trustworthy, reliable sources, preferably evidence-based ones whenever possible. Be sure to do your homework and gather as much trustworthy information from the Web as you can for your conditions(s).

You need to choose your physician(s) wisely, learning as much as possible about his/her history/record before undergoing any treatment. One way to obtain basic information on such physicians is via the Web resource—http://www.docboard.org—which contains a directory of medical boards with links to each state board's home page. Once at your state board's site, look for Physician Profiles, Search for a Physician, etc. Also, for a small fee, at—http://www.docinfo.org—you can find out if your physician(s) has been disciplined in any state—courtesy of the Federation of State Medical Boards. Inquire from others in the community about the physician's reputation.

When you go to the doctor, bring someone with you for support and to help you remember what was said. Take along a notebook with all the questions you wish to ask and obtain answers. Write all answers down in your notebook and check them for accuracy. A tape recorder is useful for this purpose as well. Do not forget to bring along all key information with you, including your medical and medication history, and Web information obtained for reference during your visit.

By using this book and advice wisely, you may benefit immeasurably.

Eugene A. DeFelice, M.D.
July 2004

Chapter 1

Searching the Web

1.1   Introduction

A number of books have been written on how to use/search the Internet/Web. You may obtain one of your choice from your local public library or bookstore and use it as an additional aid.

A number of commercial services such as AOL, MSN, Netscape, Road Runner and Yahoo, as well as others, provide easy access to the Internet/Web via your computer. If you do not have a computer, your local public, college or university library may provide one for you to use. And, if needed, your local reference librarian may provide you with assistance/instruction on how to use/search the Internet/Web as well. Should a computer not be available to you, you may use a Web TV or similar device or one of a number of handheld wireless devices now available. Once connected, a very large number of Web Resources/Websites are available for searching the Web for health information.

1.2   Selecting Appropriate Web Resources

It should be borne in mind that not all health information found on the Web can be considered trustworthy, current, comprehensive, reliable or useful. Therefore, you need to be selective and use due diligence in both searching and using health information obtained from the Web.

A reasonably prudent way to select appropriate Web Health Information Resources/Websites is to use recommended guidelines. Such guidelines are available from a number of sources such as:

- American Medical Association
  http://www.ama-assn.org
- Health on the Net Foundation
  http://www.hon.ch
- Medlineplus
  http://www.medlineplus.gov

Criteria used by different organizations in selecting reliable Web Health Information Resources/Websites vary. Nevertheless, guidelines developed by the above mentioned 3 organizations allow you to select Web Resources that may be considered to be reasonably trustworthy.

1.3　General Searching Considerations

The World Wide Web currently is estimated at well over 4 billion pages, and still growing and changing rapidly. However, one should note that Search Engines (such as Google or AlltheWeb) do not allow you to search the entire Web directly as such is not feasible at this time.

The Web is the totality of all the Web pages and documents that reside on computers, called servers, worldwide. Your computer cannot locate all these servers directly. All you can do via a search is to connect to one of a number of intermediate resources that contain selected and organized databases and Web pages. Thus, AlltheWeb, Google, and other search engines, merely allow you to search their intermediate databases/resources, and they provide a compilation of links to appropriate Web pages/information. You can then review these Web pages/links and retrieve information contained therein pertaining to your particular search.

AlltheWeb, Google and other search engines may provide you with "reasonably complete" searches of the Web. However, then you are left with the very difficult and time consuming task of reviewing up to hundreds or thousands or more Web pages/reports provided in order to determine which contain trustworthy, current, comprehensive, reliable, and useful information. Unfortunately this is usually well beyond the capability of the vast majority of readers to accomplish satisfactorily in a reasonable period of time.

In order to simplify matters for you in this regard, the author has carefully selected, personally reviewed and assembled the Author's List: Key Web Health Resources/Websites which are considered to be trustworthy and listed them alphabetically for ease of reference in Chapter 3. Each of these Web Health Resources/Websites provides a Search Site and click on Links that may be used to obtain desired information on the subject(s) you may search.

This Author's List consists chiefly of health information provided by key expert professional organizations (.org in the Web address), U.S. Government resources (.gov in the Web address), and university based sites (.edu in the Web address). Also included in the List are two key European sites, the Health On the Net Foundation in Geneva, Switzerland and the Karolinska Institute in Stockholm, Sweden. Both of these European Web Resources/Websites are considered to be among the best available and provide an international point of view in searching for trustworthy health and wellness information.

In instituting any search for health and wellness information, it is important to remember that the Internet/Web is growing rapidly and is in a constant state of flux, updating and reorganizing. Web Resources may change/modify their name and/or Website address, format, content and categorization/display of information offered.

If for any reason, the Website you have chosen doesn't work for you, search the respective Web Resource name itself. Should a problem still persist, use another Search Engine to access the Website or Web Resource in question.

Also, keep in mind that Web Resources use different methods to search the Web to compile their databases. Each Web Resource organizes/assembles information differently, some better and easier to use than others. Thus, different Web Resources/Websites, likely will provide information that may differ significantly and need to be reconciled. And, Web pages/reports/information may be removed or become unavailable on any given Web Resource/Website for a number of reasons, and substitutions of desired information from other Web Resources/Websites may become necessary.

In general, the health and wellness information obtained via the Author's List: Key Web Health Resources/Websites in Chapter 3 may be regarded as trustworthy and useful in most instances/respects but not necessarily all. Unlike medical/scientific articles published in peer review professional journals, there is no guarantee that health information obtained from any single Web Health Resource/Website may necessarily be relied upon as the "gospel". Therefore you need to be certain to select Web Resources/Websites that are appropriate for the subject being searched. Health and wellness information obtained from any one source should be compared with that from at least two other Web Health Resources/Websites and any differences reconciled whenever possible in consultation with your healthcare provider/physician. Even in the amazing world of the Web, a second and even a third opinion, may be considered worthwhile.

You also need to bear in mind that even in the case of scientific, evidence-based information from well-controlled clinical trials, there are problems in terms of what the data collected/results may mean. Clinical trial evidence necessarily is subject to interpretation and application and, as such, this is a subjective process. Everyone is biased to some degree in one way or another in obtaining, interpreting and applying information, evidence based or not. Words, phrases, statistics, conclusions, etc. mean different things to different people at different times and places, depending on "where one is coming from" so to speak. For example, even in the case of a long standing document, the Constitution of the United States, written by "great minds"—individuals, lawyers, judges, and even the Supreme Court of the United States still continue to debate, argue about, and usually have great difficulty interpreting and applying, the so-called "original intent" of the founding fathers/authors of this great document.

Nevertheless, you may have a certain degree of confidence that information obtained via the Web Resources in this book may improve your health, wellness and longevity. Therefore, become informed in order to live a healthier, happier, longer and more productive/enjoyable life.

1.4   Strategy for Successful Searching

The Author's List in Chapter 3 contains over 300 personally selected, reasonably trustworthy key US Government, medical school/center, professional organization, and European Web Resources/Websites. From this List, the Author has selected 10 of these Key Web Health Resources that are generally considered to be most useful in the vast majority of all searches. These are:

Ten Key Web Health Resources/Websites

- Key US Government Web Health Resources/Websites
  - Healthfinder
    http://www.healthfinder.gov
  - Medlineplus
    http://www.medlineplus.gov
  - National Institutes of Health
    http://www.health.nih.gov
  - National Library of Medicine
    http://www.nlm.nih.gov
  - PubMed
    http://www.ncbi.nlm.nih.gov/pubmed

- **Key Medical School/Center Health Web Resources/Websites**
    - Harvard Medical School/Consumer Health
      http://www.intellihealth.com
    - Johns Hopkins Medical Center
      http://www.hopkinsmedicine.org
    - Mayo Clinic
      http://www.mayoclinic.com

- **Key European Web Health Resources/Websites**
    - Health on the Net Foundation
      http://www.hon.ch
    - Karolinska Institute
      http://www.mic.ki.se

In most instances, you may accomplish a successful search using these Ten Key Web Health Resources following the steps below.

Step 1

In beginning your search in Step I, first familiarize yourself with the Subject List/Websites in Chapter 2. This list contains over 600 alphabetically arranged subjects and their corresponding websites.

From this Subject List, select your subject(s) and use the Search Site and Links in the corresponding Website(s) provided for the information you seek.

If for any reason you do not find your subject anywhere on the List, or if the information obtained via Step 1 is insufficient for your purpose(s) and/or requires corroboration from an additional source(s), proceed with Step 2.

Step 2

Step 2 consists of using the Healthfinder and Medlineplus Web Health Resources and their Search Sites and Links in your search.

Further searching beyond Step 2 usually is unnecessary in most instances.

Step 3

However, should you find that more information is needed to complete your search, you may obtain this from the other Key U.S. Government Health Resources, Key Medical School/Center Health Resources or Key European Web

Resources listed in the previous table. In addition, by familiarizing yourself with the full Author's List in Chapter 3, you also may find an additional Web Resource(s) that enable you to complete your search.

In case of rare diseases, disorders, or syndromes, you may find it useful to search the following Web Resources/Websites and Links directly:

- Office of Rare Diseases/National Institutes of Health
  http://www.rarediseases.info.nih.gov/ord
- Health on the Net Foundation/Rare disease
  http://www.hon.ch

Finally you may use the Search Sites of Google (http://www.google.com) and/or AlltheWeb (http://www.alltheweb.com) to obtain a "reasonably complete" search of "all" available information on the Web contained in their databases.

1.4.1 Key US Government Web Health Resources/Websites

1.4.1.1 Healthfinder
http://www.healthfinder.gov

Healthfinder was developed in 1997 by the US Department of Health and Human Services (http://www.os.dhhs.gov) in conjunction with other Federal Agencies. It is recognized as a key resource in finding US Government health, wellness, and services information on the Web. Healthfinder has links to carefully selected information and Websites from over 1800 health related organizations. It is coordinated by the Office of Disease Prevention and Health Promotion (http://www.od.nih.gov) with participation of a Steering Committee composed of: 1) representatives of the federal agencies (whose information is used), 2) non-federal consumer health information specialists, 3) librarians, and 4) others actively engaged in the provision or use of online consumer health information.

Healthfinder represents a "virtual library" of reliable health information that is hand picked from US government agencies, non profit organizations, and medical schools/universities/centers.

Health information on this Website is organized into the following categories:

- **Health Library**—provides health information A to Z on prevention and wellness, diseases and conditions, alternative medicine, medical dictionaries, medical encyclopedias, journals, prescription drug information, and more.
- **Just for You**—covers a number of health subjects organized for men and women, by age, for kids to seniors, by race and ethnicity, and for parents, caregivers, healthcare professionals and others.

- **Health Care**—includes information about doctors, dentists, public clinics, hospitals, long term care, support groups, nursing homes, health insurance, prescription drugs, health fraud, Medicare, Medicaid, and medical privacy.
- **Directory of Healthfinder Organizations**—lists carefully selected health information Websites from government agencies, clearinghouses, non profit organizations, and medical schools/universities/centers. You may search these by name, browse by topic or consult an alphabetical list of organizations for additional information.
- **Health News**—provides a discussion of the latest key health news on a variety of subjects.

1.4.1.2 Medlineplus
http://www.medlineplus.gov

Medlineplus is a service of the National Library of Medicine (http://www.nlm.nih.gov), the world's largest medical library, and the National Institutes of Health (http://www.nih.gov), a trusted source of medical information, utilizing their online databases involving over 14 million citations. Medlineplus does not accept any advertising on their Website nor do they endorse any company product. It provides summaries of information and references as well as links to further information.

Health information is made available in the following formats:

- **Health Topics**—presenting over 600 subjects/topics on conditions and diseases and wellness
- **Drug Information**—regarding prescription and over the counter medicines
- **Medical Encyclopedia**—covering numerous conditions, diseases, and other subjects including pictures and diagrams
- **Dictionary**—providing spellings and definitions of medical words/items
- **News**—describing important health news from the past 30 day period
- **Directories**—enabling the reader to find doctors, dentists, and hospitals
- **Other Resources**—lists of local libraries, professional health organizations, international sites and more
- **Interactive Tutorials**—slide shows with sound and pictures on key health subjects
- **Clinical Trials.gov**—covers studies for new drugs and treatments
- **NIH Senior Health**—information for older adults
- **Links**—to the National Library of Medicine, National Institutes of Health, and the Department of Health and Human Services for additional information.

Health Topics—provides an A to Z alphabetical list that helps you find your subject of interest. You may click on the first letter to gain access to your subject/information desired. In addition, you can click on the appropriate subject, or inclusive group, from lists provided including:

1. **Disorders and Conditions/Body Locations and Systems**
   - Blood/Lymphatic Systems
   - Bones, Joints and Muscles
   - Brain and Nervous System
   - Cancer
   - Complementary/Alternative Therapies
   - Digestive System
   - Ear, Nose and Throat
   - Endocrine System (Hormones)
   - Eyes and Vision
   - Genetics/Birth Defects
   - Heart and Circulation
   - Immune System/AIDS
   - Infections
   - Injuries and Wounds
   - Kidneys and Urinary System
   - Lungs and Breathing
   - Mental Health and Behavior
   - Mouth and Teeth
   - Poisoning, Toxicology, and Environmental Health
   - Pregnancy and Reproduction
   - Skin, Hair and Nails
   - Substance Abuse
   - Symptoms and Manifestations

2. **Demographic Groups**
   - Child and Teen Health
   - Men's Health
   - Population Groups
   - Senior's Health
   - Women's Health

3. **Health and Wellness**
   - Food, Nutrition and Metabolism
   - Health System

- Safety
- Sexual Health
- Social/Family Issues
- Wellness and Lifestyle

1.4.1.3 National Institutes of Health
   http://www.health.nih.gov

The National Institutes of Health is composed of 27 Institutes and Centers, and is regarded as the premier international research institution and repository for medical/health information in the world.

In searching a health subject at this site, the system automatically refers you to information contained at the appropriate NIH Institute or Center concerned.

Health Information—provides the following click on categories/links:

- **Center for Drug Evaluation and Research**—drug information for consumers from the FDA
- **Clinical Trials**—provides information on medical studies around the USA
- **Drug Information**—information guide on over 9,000 medications
- **Healthfinder**—a health resource maintained by the Department of Health and Human Services
- **Medlineplus**—a health database maintained by NIH's National Library of Medicine

Both Healthfinder and Medlineplus provide click on links to the US National Library of Medicine, the World's largest medical library and creator of Medline/PubMed.

Search for a Health Topic—allows you to search for additional information

You may click on and **Browse Health Topics Alphabetically** by the first subject letter A to Z, or click on **See All Topics.**

Search Your Health Topic—in one of the following categories:
1. **Body Locations/Systems**
- Blood/Lymphatic System
- Bones, Joints and Muscles
- Brain and Nervous system
- Digestive System
- Ear, Nose and Throat

- Endocrine System (Hormones)
- Eyes and Vision
- Heart and Circulation
- Immune System
- Kidney and Urinary System
- Lungs and Breathing
- Mental Health and Behavior
- Mouth and Teeth
- Pregnancy and Reproduction
- Skin, Hair and Nails
2. **Procedures**
- Procedures and Therapies
- Symptoms and Manifestations
3. **Common Conditions/Diseases**
- Cancers
- Genetics/Birth defects
- Infections
- Injuries and Wounds
4. **Health and Wellness**
- Environmental Health
- Substance Abuse
- Food, Nutrition and Metabolism
- Safety
- Sexual Health
- Social/Family Issues
- Wellness and Lifestyle
5. **Demographic Groups**
- Child and Teen Health
- Men's Health
- Population Groups
- Senior's Health
- Women's Health

1.4.1.4 National Library of Medicine
http://www.nlm.nih.gov

Health Information at the National Library of Medicine is provided by Medline/PubMed, Medlineplus and NLM Gateway plus other channels.

Additional information also is available via the NLM **Search Site**.

Health Information—organized into the following click on categories:
- **Medlineplus**—provides answers to your health questions/subjects search
- **Medline/PubMed**—abstracts and references from 4600 biomedical journals
- **Clinical Trials.gov**—about clinical research studies and possible participation therein
- **Dirline**—directory of health organizations
- **Locatorplus**—catalog of books, journals and audiovisuals
- **NIH Senior Health**—health information for older adults
- **NLM Gateway**–interface that searches multiple NLM retrieval systems
- **PubMed Central**—digital archive of life sciences journal literature
- **Toxnet**—toxicology, environmental health, and hazardous chemicals information
- **ToxTown**—guide to commonly encountered toxic substances, your health and the environment.

Click on Links—available for information on:
- **AIDS/HIV**
- **Bioethics**
- **Cancer**
- **Chemical Substances**
- **Health Services Research and Health Care Technology**
- **History of Medicine**
- **Malaria**
- **Molecular Biology/Genetics**
- **Public Health**
- **Space Life Sciences**
- **Toxicology and Environmental Health**

Other links are provided for information about all NLM Databases and Electronic Information Resources, National Institutes of Health and the Department of Health and Human Services.

- **Call the NIH**—toll-free information lines listed by health condition.
- **Database/Toll Free Numbers**—for health organizations around the USA
- **Library References**—including:
  - **PubMed**—comprehensive database of article titles, abstracts and references
  - **Combined Health Information Database**—for article titles and abstracts
  - **International Bibliographic Information on Dietary Supplements (IBIDs)**—article titles focused on dietary supplements.

- Special Programs—including:
  - **Complementary and Alternative Medicine**—research on adjunct therapies
  - **Rare Diseases**—research, clinical trials, and patient support groups
  - **Women's Health**—health issues specific to women
  - **Minority Health**—health status of minority Americans
  - **Behavorial and Social Sciences**—social science research across NIH
  - **Bioethics Resources**—medical, healthcare, and research ethics
  - **NIH Clinical Alerts**—findings from NIH funded clinical trials
  - **Consumer Development Program**—updates on medical practice
- Other Health Agencies—including:
  - **Centers for Disease Control and Prevention (CDC)**—protecting the public health
  - **Food and Drug Administration (FDA)**—product approvals and safety alerts
  - **Agency for Healthcare Research and Quality**—insurance, prescription and patient information

1.4.1.5   PubMed
http://www.ncbi.nlm.nih.gov/pubmed

PubMed is a service of the National Library of Medicine and includes over 14 million citations for biomedical articles dating back to the 1950s. It makes available a comprehensive database of published article titles and abstracts plus references on subjects searched.

Citations are from **Medline** and additional life science journals.

PubMed includes links to other key Websites that provide full text articles as well as other related information resources.

A **Search Site** is provided for additional information, or you may click on the **Preview/Index** link for advanced searching.

Health and Wellness Information—categorized as follows:
- **PubMed Services**—includes click on links for:
  - Batch Citation Matcher
  - Clinical Queries
  - Journals Database
  - Linkout
  - MeSH Database
  - Single Citation Matcher
- **Related Resources**–includes click on sites for:
  - Clinical Alerts
  - Clinical Trials.gov

- Consumer Health
- New Global NCBI Search Engine
- NLM Gateway
- Order Documents
- PubMed Central
- Toxnet

PubMed includes key links to Websites providing full text articles as well as other related resources.

1.4.2 Key Medical School/Center Web Health Resources/Websites

1.4.2.1 Harvard Medical School/Consumer Health http://www.intellihealth.com

This Website features **Harvard Medical School's Consumer Health** Information.

In August 2000, Harvard Medical School, one of the world's preeminent health institutions, became the flagship medical content partner of Intellihealth. A core editorial faculty of 14 physicians and one pharmacist works closely with Intellihealth to create content, review articles and other information for clinical accuracy and relevance. Numerous contributing editors on the Harvard Medical School faculty work with the core faculty to maintain standards for all health information content.

Information Sites are featured on:
- Ask the Expert
- Communities/Chats
- Dental Health
- Drug Resource Center
- Health Commentaries
- Interactive Tools
- Today's News
- **Disease and Conditions A to Z**
- **Healthy Lifestyle**
  - Complementary and Alternative Medicine
  - Fitness
  - Nutrition
  - Weight Management
  - Workplace Health

- **Your Health**
  - Children's Health
  - Men's Health
  - Senior's Health
  - Women's Health
- **Look It Up**
  - Drug Resource Center
  - Health A to Z
  - Medical Dictionary
- **Enter a Drug Name Search Site**
- **Enter a Subject/Term Search Site**

1.4.2.2 Johns Hopkins University Medical Center
http://www.hopkinsmedicine.org

Johns Hopkins University Medical Center has provided international leadership in the education of physicians, medical scientists, in biomedical research, and in the application of medical knowledge to sustain health since the opening of Johns Hopkins Hospital in 1889.

Today, Johns Hopkins is a growing, evolving healthcare enterprise. Its Executive Dean, Elias Zerhouni, was selected by President George W. Bush to run the nation's major research engine, the National Institutes of Health. In addition, once again Johns Hopkins was named the No. 1 hospital in the United States and the medical school was named one of the best in the nation—also being ranked No. 1 in receipt of NIH research dollars.

Johns Hopkins is regarded as providing trustworthy, current, useful health information for both patients/consumers and health professionals.

Health Information click on sites include:
- Allergy and Asthma
- Arthritis
- Bladder, Kidney and Liver Disorders
  - Bladder cancer
  - Liver transplants
  - Urological diseases
- Blood Disorders
- Bones, Joints and Muscles
  - Bone Marrow Transplant
  - Sports medicine

- Cancer
- Children's Health
- Diabetes
- Digestive Disorders
  - Gallbladder and Bile Duct Cancer
- Ears, Nose and Throat
  - Barrett's Esophagus
- Eye and Vision Disorders
- Heart and Circulatory System
  - Heart Transplants
- Infectious Disease
  - AIDS/HIV
  - Tuberculosis
- Lung and Breathing Disorders
  - Lung Transplants
- Mental Health
- Neurological Disease
  - ALS (Lou Gehrig's Disease)
  - Alzheimer's Disease
  - Epilepsy Center
  - Parkinson's Disease Research Center
  - Restless Leg Syndrome
- Skin Disorders
- Thyroid and Hormonal Disorders
  - Hypophysitis
- Women's Health
  - Cervical Dysplasia
  - Johns Hopkins Breast Center
  - Kelly G. Ripken Program
  - Ovarian Cancer
- Subject Search Site

1.4.2.3 Mayo Clinic
http://www.mayoclinic.com

The **Mayo Clinic** is an exemplary non profit organization with over 2000 physicians and 35,000 allied health staff, scientists, researchers, and other professionals. Its mission is to empower people to manage their own health, accomplishing this by providing health information and tools that reflect the expertise and standard of excellence of the Mayo Clinic. A team of Web publishing professionals and medical experts is involved in this effort providing current, comprehensive, reliable and useful health information through their database and key links to other resources.

Health Information is provided in both English and Spanish languages.

Diseases and Conditions features click on sites for:

- **A to Z List**—all about a disease or condition in one comprehensive overview
- **Disease and Conditions Centers**—select a center for a collection of information and tools to help you manage your condition
- **Health Decision Guides**—tools to help you weigh the pros and cons of different options and choose which approach is best for you. Click on site examples include:
  - Adjuvant Therapy for Breast Cancer
  - Children's Middle Ear Infection
  - Colorectal Cancer Screening
  - Early Stage Breast Cancer
  - Early Stage Prostate Cancer
  - Herniated disk
  - Knee Injuries
  - Uterine Fibroids
- **Drug Search**—allows you to browse drugs by name or category and find information on prescription and over the counter drugs from A-Z. Included is information on:
  - General Information About the Use of Medicines
  - Avoiding Medicine Mishaps: Tips Against Tampering
  - Getting the Most Out of Your Medicine
  - About the Medicine You Are Taking
  - Search Site—Enter a Drug Name
- **Health Tools**—provides click on sites for:
  - Self-assessments
    - Depression Self Assessment
    - Personal Health Scorecard
  - Calculators
    - BMI Calculator
    - Heart Disease Risk Calculator
    - Skin Type Calculator
    - Target Heart Rate Calculator

- **Healthy Living Centers**—features click on sites for:
  - Baby's Health
  - Children's Health
  - Complementary and Alternative Medicine
  - Fitness and Sports Medicine
  - Food and Nutrition
  - Men's Health
  - Pregnancy
  - Senior Health
  - Women's Health
  - Working Life

1.4.3 Key European Web Health Resources/Websites

1.4.3.1 Health on the Net Foundation
http://www.hon.ch

HON, established in 1995, is one of the most respected non profit Web Resources providing health information on the Web. It is a Swiss foundation operating out of Geneva, Switzerland in close cooperation with the University Hospitals of Geneva and the Swiss Institute of Bioinformatics. HON's distinguished guiding council members and Web team hail from several European countries and the USA.

Distinguishing features of this web resource are two widely used medical search tools, MedHunt and HONSelect.

The HON Code of Conduct provides leadership in establishing ethical standards for Website providers around the world.

Health information is provided by site source and location, degree of relevance to subject, and date. It is provided in English and other languages. Click on sites include:

- **Daily News**—latest health news from selected trustworthy sources
- **HON Media**—top selection of illustrations representing over 1400 subjects
- **HON Project**—discusses projects initiated by HON to help build the medical community of the Internet/Web, MedHunt, HONselect, and the HON Code of Conduct (HON Code) are among HON services that actively promote effective internet use and seek to demonstrate best-in-class implementation and application. MedHunt consists of a specialized search engine designed to locate Internet/Web information related to a given medical and health domain. HON select is the first assisted search facility that integrates heterogeneous databases to offer users a full assortment of

healthcare information and resources available on the Web. HON Code is an authoritative set of voluntary guidelines designed to raise the quality of Web based medical and health information. The HON Code today is the most widely endorsed set of ethical guidelines for Website developers in the medical and health domains.

- **HONcode Toolbar**—for health information you can trust
- **HONDossier**—health topics which deserve special attention with special in-depth reports on such subjects as:
  - Aging
  - Allergy Glossary
  - Hepatitis B
  - Mother and Child
  - Rare Disease
  - Stop Smoking
  - Vision and Eyecare FAQ
- **HONselect**—33,000 medical definitions and trustworthy sources in 5 languages
- **MedHunt**—search full text of over 90,000 worldwide medical documents
- **Medical Professionals**
- **Medline/PubMed/National Library of Medicine USA**—click on links to these key Web Health Resources
- **Patients/Individuals**
- **Search Site**—to retrieve "trustworthy" medical documents/reports
- **Web Publishers**

1.4.3.2 Karolinska Institute
http://www.mic.ki.se

The **Karolinska Institute** in Stockholm is Sweden's only university for medicine. It accounts for around 40% of all the medical research at universities throughout the country and is Sweden's largest medical library.

A Search Site is provided for MeSH classified Web Health Resources for both the general public, patients and healthcare professionals.

MeSH—Medical Subject Headings—is the US National Library of Medicine's controlled vocabulary used to index and catalogue bibliographic and other types of biomedical information. You may use the MeSH to accomplish your subject search for desired information. Also you may click on alphabetical list of Disease/Disorders option to obtain information desired.

Users are advised to discuss results of their health and wellness searches with their healthcare provider/physicians before reaching any definitive conclusions regarding information obtained.

1.4.4 Prescription/OTC Drug Information

You may obtain prescription/OTC drug information, in most instances, by using a Search Engine such as Google or AlltheWeb and searching as follows:
- type in http://www. and then enter the name of the drug followed by .com

For example, if you are looking for information on the cholesterol/triglyceride lowering drug, Zocor, or the blood pressure lowering agent, Diovan, you may search respectively as follows:
For Zocor
- http://www.zocor.com
For Diovan
- http://www.diovan.com

In most cases this will allow you to obtain not only significant detailed information on the drug(s) of interest but also the disorders(s) indicated—for both patients/consumers and health professionals/physicians.

In addition, you also may go to the Subject List in Chapter 2 and search the Websites given under Prescription/OTC Drug Information, namely:
- http://www.druginfonet.com
- http://www.fda.gov
- http://www.rxlist.com

Such searches should provide you with most, if not all the information you are seeking, in most cases.

Additional medication information is available by searching the drug name in key US government, medical school/center, and European Web Health Resources listed in 1.4.1-1.4.3.2, or Google (http://www.google.com) or AlltheWeb (http://www.alltheweb.com).

Chapter 2

Alphabetical List of Subjects/Websites

2.1   Abdominal Disorders to Autoimmune Disease

- Abdominal Disorders
  - http://www.aafp.org
  - http://www.acg.gi.org
  - http://www.acponline.org
  - http://www.gastro.org
- Abortion
  - http://www.nric.org
  - http://www.ppfa.org
- Abrasions
  - http://www.aad.org
  - http://www.aafp.org
- Acne
  - http://www.aad.org
  - http://www.aafp.org
  - http://www.niams.nih.gov
- Acoustic Neuroma
  - http://www.aan.com
  - http://www.anausa.org
  - http://www.audiology.org

- Acromegaly
  - http://www.aan.com
  - http://www.ninds.nih.gov
- Actinic Skin Keratosis
  - http://www.aad.org
  - http://www.aafp.org
- Acupuncture
  - http://www.acuall.org
  - http://www.nccam.nih.gov
- Addiction
  - http://www.ncadd.net
  - http://www.ncpgambling.org
  - http://www.niaaa.nih.gov
  - http://www.nida.nih.gov
  - http://www.nmha.org
- Addison Disease
  - http://www.aace.com/college
  - http://www.acponline.org
  - http://www.endo-society.org
  - http://www.medhelp.org/nadf
- Aging
  - http://www.aoa.dhhs.gov
  - http://www.cdc.gov
  - http://www.geron.org
  - http://www.hcoa.org
  - http://www.nia.nih.gov
- Agranulocytosis
  - http://www.aafp.org
  - http://www.acponline.org
  - http://www.healthcare.ucla.edu
  - http://www.hematology.org
  - http://www.nhlbi.nih.gov
- AIDS/HIV
  - http://www.ama-assn.org
  - http://www.cdc.gov
  - http://www.niaid.nih.gov
- Air Pollution/Air Borne Diseases
  - http://www.cdc.gov
  - http://www.lungusa.org

- Albinism
  - http://www.aad.org
  - http://www.medhelp.org
  - http://www.niams.nih.gov
  - http://www.noah-health.org
- Alcoholism/Alcoholics Anonymous
  - http://www.alcoholics-anonymous.org
  - http://www.ncadd.net
  - http://www.niaaa.nih.gov
  - http://www.nmha.org
  - http://www.rational.org
- Allergy/Children and Adults
  - http://www.aaaai.org
  - http://www.aafa.org
  - http://www.aap.org
  - http://www.allergy.mcg.edu
  - http://www.medhelp.org
  - http://www.niaid.nih.gov
- Alopecia/Hair Loss
  - http://www.aad.org
  - http://www.aafp.org
  - http://www.alopeciaareata.com
  - http://www.medhelp.org
- Alternative/Complementary Medicine
  - http://www.bcm.tmc.edu
  - http://www.herbalgram.org
  - http://www.nccam.nih.gov
  - http://www.pitt.edu/~cbw.altm.html
- Alzheimer's Disease
  - http://www.alz.org
  - http://www.alzheimers.org
  - http://www.alzheimers-research.org
  - http://www.nmha.org
- Amblyopia/Lazy Eye Syndrome
  - http://www.aao.org
  - http://www.nei.nih.gov
  - http://www.preventblindness.org

- **Amenorrhea**
  - http://www.aafp.org
  - http://www.acog.org
  - http://www.mc.vanderbilt.edu
- **Amyotropic Lateral Sclerosis**
  - http://www.aan.com
  - http://www.clevelandclinic.org
  - http://www.ninds.nih.gov
- **Angioneuotic Edema/Hives**
  - http://www.aaaai.org
  - http://www.allergy.mcg.edu
  - http://www.medhelp.org
- **Ankylosing Spondylitis**
  - http://www.acponline.org
  - http://www.arthritis.org
  - http://www.niams.nih.gov
  - http://www.rhematology.org
- **Anal Abscess/Fissure**
  - http://www.aafp.org
  - http://www.fascrs.org
- **Anaphylaxis**
  - http://www.aaaai.org
  - http://www.medhelp.org
- **Anemia**
  - http://www.aafp.org
  - http://www.aarda.org
  - http://www.hematology.org
  - http://www.irondisorders.org
  - http://www.nhlbi.gov
- **Anesthesia**
  - http://www.asahq.org
  - http://www.medhelp.org
  - http://www.webmd.com
- **Aneurysm**
  - http://www.aans.org
  - http://www.acc.org
  - http://www.americanheart.org
  - http://www.nhlbi.nih.gov

- **Angina Pectoris**
  - http://www.aafp.org
  - http://www.acc.org
  - http://www.americanheart.org
  - http://www.nhlbi.nih.gov
- **Angiography**
  - http://www.acc.org
  - http://www.nhlbi.nih.org
  - http://www.scvir.org
- **Angioplasty/Stents**
  - http://www.acc.org
  - http://www.nhlbi.gov
  - http://www.scvir.org
- **Animal to Human Disease**
  - http://www.aafp.org
  - http://www.acponline.org
  - http://www.aphl.org
  - http://www.cdc.gov
  - http://www.who.int
- **Anorexia/Loss of Appetite**
  - http://www.aafp.org
  - http://www.acponline.org
- **Anorexia Nervosa**
  - http://www.aafp.org
  - http://www.anad.org
  - http://www.nimh.nih.gov
  - http://www.nmha.org
- **Anthrax**
  - http://www.cdc.gov
  - http://www.niaid.nih.gov
- **Anxiety States**
  - http://www.mentalhelp.net
  - http://www.nimh.nih.gov
  - http://www.nmha.org
- **Aortic Valve Disease/Replacement**
  - http://www.acc.org
  - http://www.americanheart.org
  - http://www.nhlbi.nih.gov
  - http://www.sts.org

- Aphasia
  - http://www.aan.org
  - http://www.ninds.nih.gov
  - http://www.stroke.org
- Aphthous Stomatis/Mouth Ulcer
  - http://www.aafp.org
  - http://www.aahcfp.org
  - http://www.allergy.mcg.edu
  - http://www.entnet.org
- Appendicitis
  - http://www.aafp.org
  - http://www.facs.org
  - http://www.niddk.nih.gov
  - http://www.yoursurgery.com
- Appetite Loss/Anorexia
  - http://www.aafp.org
  - http://www.healthcare.ucla.edu
- Arrhythmia/Cardiac
  - http://www.aafp.org
  - http://www.acc.org
  - http://www.americanheart.org
  - http://www.nhlbi.nih.gov
- Arsenic Poisoning
  - http://www.aafp.org
  - http://www.aapcc.org
  - http://www.cdc.gov
- Arthritis/Arthralgia
  - http://www.aafp.org
  - http://www.arthritis.org
  - http://www.niams.nih.gov
- Arthropathy
  - http://www.aofas.org
  - http://www.niams.nih.gov
- Arthroscopy
  - http://www.aaos.org
  - http://www.aofas.org
- Asbestosis
  - http://www.cdc.gov
  - http://www.chestnut.org
  - http://www.lungusa.org

- **Ascites**
  - http://www.aafp.org
  - http://www.acg.gi.org
  - http://www.acponline.org
  - http://www.liverfoundation.org
- **Asperger's Syndrome**
  - http://www.aan.com
  - http://www.medhelp.org
  - http://www.ninds.nih.gov
- **Asthma**
  - http://www.aaaai.org
  - http://www.aafp.org
  - http://www.chestnet.org
  - http://www.nhbli.nih.gov
- **Ataxia**
  - http://www.aan.org
  - http://www.acponline.org
  - http://www.ataxia.org
- **Athlete's Foot/Tinea Pedis**
  - http://www.aad.org
  - http://www.aafp.org
  - http://www.aap.org
- **Athererosclerosis**
  - http://www.aafp.org
  - http://www.acc.org
  - http://www.acponline.org
  - http://www.americanheart.org
- **Atmospheric Pollution/Disease**
  - http://www.acpm.org
  - http://www.aphl.org
  - http://www.cdc.gov
  - http://www.lungsusa.org
  - http;//www.niehs.nih.org
- **Atrial Fibrillation**
  - http://www.acc.org
  - http://www.americanheart.org
  - http://www.nhlbi.nih.gov

- Attention Deficit/Hyperactivity Disorder
  - http://www.aafp.org
  - http://www.aap.org
  - http://www.chadd.org
  - http://www.nimh.nih.gov
  - http://www.nmha.org
- Autism
  - http://www.nacd.org
  - http://www.niehd.nih.gov
  - http://www.nimh.nih.gov
  - http://www.nmha.org
- Autoimmune Disease
  - http://www.aai.org
  - http://www.aarda.org
  - http://www.healthcare.ucla.edu
  - http://www.niaid.nih.gov

2.2   Back/Spine Problems to Bursitis

- Back/Spine Problems
  - http://www.aafp.org
  - http://www.aanos.org
  - http://www.aans.org
  - http://www.arthritis.org
  - http://www.backpainreliefonline.com
  - http://www.niams.nih.gov
- Balance Disorders/Falls
  - http://www.aafp.org
  - http://www.aan.org
  - http://www.americangeriatrics.org
  - http://www.auanet.org
  - http://www.healthcare.ucla.edu
- Balantitis
  - http://www.aafp.org
  - http://www.auanet.org
- Barrett's Esophagus
  - http://www.acg.gi.org
  - http://www.gastro.org
  - http://www.niddk.nih.gov

- Bartholin Cyst
  - http://www.aafp.org
  - http://www.medhelp.org
- Behcet's Syndrome
  - http://www.acponline.org
  - http://www.healthsystem.virginia.edu
  - http://www.niams.nih.gov
  - http://www.noah-health.org
  - http://www.mc.vanderbilt.edu
- Bell's Facial Palsy
  - http://www.aan.com
  - http://www.entnet.org
  - http://www.healthsystem.virginia.edu
  - http://www.noah-health.org
- Bird/Avian Flu
  - http://www.aafp.org
  - http://www.acponline.org
  - http://www.aphl.org
  - http://www.cdc.gov
  - http://www.niaid.nih.gov
  - http://www.nfid.org
- Birth Defects
  - http://www.aap.org
  - http://www.acog.org
  - http://www.cleftpalate-craniofacial.org
  - http://www.kidshealth.org
  - http://www.nacd.org
  - http://www.nichd.nih.gov
- Birthmarks
  - http://www.aad.org
  - http://www.aafp.org
  - http://www.aap.org
  - http://www.acog.org
- Bladder Cancer
  - http://www.afud.org
  - http://www.cancer.gov
  - http://www.niddk.nih.gov
- Bleeding Gums
  - http://www.aafp.org
  - http://www.ada.org

- **Blepharitis/Eyelid Infection**
  - http://www.aafp.org
  - http://www.aao.org
  - http://www.nei.nih.gov
- **Blood Banks**
  - http://www.aabb.org
  - http://www.nhlbi.nih.gov
- **Blood/Bleeding Disorders**
  - http://www.aafp.org
  - http://www.acponline.org
  - http://www.aspho.org
  - http://www.healthcare.ucla.edu
  - http://www.hematology.org
  - http://www.nhlbi.nih.gov
- **Blood in Stool/Melena**
  - http://www.aafp.org
  - http://www.acg.gi.org
  - http://www.gastro.org
- **Blood Transfusions**
  - http;//www.aabb.org
  - http://www.americansblood.org
  - http://www.nhlbi.nih.gov
- **Boil/Carbuncle/Furuncle**
  - http://www.aad.org
  - http://www.aafp.org
- **Bone/Joint Disease/Heel Spur**
  - http://www.aaos.org
  - http://www.apma.org
  - http://www.arthritis.org
  - http://www.medhelp.org
  - http://www.niams.nih.org
- **Bone Marrow Transplant**
  - http://www.aai.org
  - http://www.bmnews.org
  - http://www.bmtinfonet.org
  - http://www.healthcare.ucla.edu
  - http://www.healthsystem.virginia.edu
- **Botulism**
  - http://www.aafp.org
  - http://www.cdc.gov

- **Bowel Incontinence**
  - http://www.aafp.org
  - http://www.fascrs.org
- **Brain Disorders**
  - http://www.aan.com
  - http://www.ninds.nih.gov
- **Brain Injury**
  - http://www.aan.com
  - http://www.biausa.org
  - http://www.ninds.nih.gov
- **Brain Hemorrhage**
  - http://www.aafp.org
  - http://www.aan.org
  - http://www.acponline.org
  - http://www.ninds.nih.gov
- **Brain Scan**
  - http://www.aahcfp.org
  - http://www.aans.com
  - http://www.acr.org
- **Breast Cancer**
  - http://www.acog.org
  - http://www.bcaction.org
  - http://www.breast-cancer-research.com
  - http://www.cancer.gov
  - http://www.komen.org
  - http://www.oncolink.org
- **Breast Disease**
  - http://www.acog.org
  - http://www.4women.org
  - http://www.womens_health.org
  - http://www.womenshealthmatters.ca
- **Breast Feeding**
  - http://www.aafp.org
  - http://www.aap.org
  - http://www.acog.org
  - http://www.ama-assn.org
  - http://www.who.int
- **Breast Implants**
  - http://www.acog.org
  - http://www.fda.gov

- Breast Self-Examination
  - http://www.4women.org
  - http://www.komen.org
  - http://www.womens_health.org
  - http://www.womenshealthmatters.ca
- Bronchiectasis
  - http://www.aafp.org
  - http://www.chestnet.org
  - http://www.lungusa.org
  - http://www.nhlbi.nih.gov
- Bronchitis
  - http://www.aafp.org
  - http://www.aafs.org
  - http://www.chestnet.org
  - http://www.lungusa.org
- Bronchoscopy
  - http://www.chestnet.org
  - http://www.lungusa.org
- Brucellosis
  - http://www.cdc.gov
  - http://www.niaid.nih.gov
- Bruise/Contusion
  - http://www.aad.org
  - http://www.aafp.org
- Bulimia
  - http://www.anad.org
  - http://www.eatingdisorders.org
  - http://www.nimh.nih.gov
  - http://www.nmha.org
- Bundle Branch Block
  - http://www.acc.org.
  - http://www.americanheart.org
  - http://www.nhlbi.nih.gov
- Bunion/Bunionette
  - http://www.aafp.org
  - http://www.apma.org
- Burns
  - http://www.aafp.org
  - http://www.cdc.gov
  - http://www.niams.nih.gov

- Bursitis
  - http://www.aafp.org
  - http://www.arthritis.org
  - http://www.niams.nih.gov

2.3   Cancer to Cystocele

- Cancer/Prevention
  - http://www.acs.org
  - http://www.acpm.org
  - http://www.asco.org
  - http://www.aspho.org
  - http://www.aspo.org
  - http://www.cancer.gov
  - http://www.cancer.org
  - http://www.cancercare.org
  - http://www.cdc.gov
  - http://www.cytopathology.org
  - http://www.mcw.edu
  - http://www.ons.org
  - http://www.who.int
- Candidiasis
  - http://www.aafp.org
  - http://www.acog.org
- Cardiac Arrest
  - http://www.acc.org
  - http://www.acep.com
  - http://www.americanheart.org
  - http://www.nhlbi.nih.gov
- Cardiology
  - http://www.acc.org
  - http://www.americanheart.org
  - http://www.medhelp.org
- Cardiomegaly
  - http://www.acc.org
  - http://www.americanheart.org
  - http://www.nhlbi.nih.gov

- Cardiomyopathy
  - http://www.acc.org
  - http://www.healthcare.ucla.edu
  - http://www.nhlbi.nih.gov
- Cardiovascular Disease/Prevention
  - http://www.acc.org
  - http://www.acpm.org
  - http://www.americanheart.org
  - http://www.nhlbi.nih.gov
- Caregivers
  - http://www.ama-assn.org
  - http://www.healthfinder.gov
  - http://www.medlineplus.gov
  - http://www.nfcacares.org
- Carotid Bruit
  - http://www.acc.org
  - http://www.americanheart.org
  - http://www.nhlbi.nih.gov
- Carpal Tunnel Syndrome
  - http://www.aafp.org
  - http://www.aans.org
- Cat Scratch Fever
  - http://www.aapf.org
  - http://www.cdc.gov
  - http://www.niaid.nih.gov
- Cataracts
  - http://www.aao.org
  - http://www.ascrs.org
  - http://www.nei.nih.gov
- Celiac Disease
  - http://www.celiac.org
  - http://www.csaceliacs.org
- Cellulitis
  - http://www.aad.org
  - http://www.aafp.org
  - http://www.acponline.org

- Cerebral Palsy
  - http://www.aacpdm.org
  - http://www.aap.org
  - http://www.ucpa.org
- Cerebrovascular Disease
  - http://www.aafp.org
  - http://www.aans.org
  - http://www.acponline.org
  - http://www.americanheart.org
  - http://www.cdc.gov
  - http://www.americangeriatrics.org
  - http://www.nhlbi.nih.gov
- Cervical Disc/Neck Disorder
  - http://www.aafp.org
  - http://www.aans.org
  - http://www.aaos.org
  - http://www.arthritis.org
  - http://www.entnet.org
- Cervical/Uterine Disease
  - http://www.aafp.org
  - http://www.acog.org
  - http://www.4women.org
  - http://www.healthywomen.org
- Chalazion
  - http://www.aafp.org
  - http://www.aao.org
- Chemical Skin Peeling
  - http://www.aad.org
  - http://www.aafp.org
  - http://www.asds-net.og
- Chest Diseases
  - http://www.chestnet.org
  - http://www.lungusa.org
  - http://www.medhelp.org
- Chest Pain
  - http://www.aafp.org
  - http://www.acponline.org
  - http://www.chestnet.org

- Chickenpox/Varicella/Vaccination
  - http://www.aafp.org
  - http://www.aap.org
  - http://www.cdc.gov
- Child Abuse
  - http://www.aacap.org
  - http://www.aafp.org
  - http://www.aap.org
  - http://www.cdc.gov
  - http://www.kidshealth.org
  - http://www.nimh.nih.gov
- Child/Adolescent Mental Health
  - http://www.aacap.org
  - http://www.aap.org
  - http://www.nimh.nih.gov
- Childbirth
  - http://www.aafp.org
  - http://www.acog.org
  - http://www.childbirth.org
  - http://www.who.int
- Child Health/Development
  - http://www.aacap.org
  - http://www.aacpdm.org
  - http://www.aap.org
  - http://www.aafp.org
  - http://www.adolescenthealth.org
  - http://www.kidshealth.org
  - http://www.nacd.org
  - http://www.nichd.nih.gov
  - http://www.nidcr.nih.gov
- Cholera
  - http://www.aphl.org
  - http://www.cdc.gov
  - http://www.niaid.nih.gov
- Chondromalacia
  - http://www.arthritis.org
  - http://www.nacd.org
  - http://www.niams.nih.gov

- **Chronic Disease Prevention**
  - http://www.acpm.org
  - http://www.cdc.gov/nccdphp/dnpa
  - http://www.od.nih.gov
- **Chronic Obstructive Pulmonary Disease**
  - http://www.chestnet.org
  - http://www.lungusa.org
  - http://www.nhlbi.nih.gov
- **Cirrhosis**
  - http://www.aafp.org
  - http://www.liver.org
  - http://www.liverfoundation.org
  - http://www.niddk.nih.gov
- **Claudication/Intermittent**
  - http://www.aafp.org
  - http://www.acponline.org
- **Cleft Palate/Lip**
  - http://www.cleft.org
  - http://www.cleftpalate-craniofacial.org
  - http://www.nichd.nih.gov
  - http://www.nidcr.nih.gov
  - http://www.plasticsurgery.org
- **Clinical Practice Guidelines**
  - http://www.acc.org
  - http://www.acponline.org
  - http://www.ama-assn.org
  - http://www.americanheart.org
  - http://www.asim.org
  - http://www.cdc.gov
  - http://www.guideline.gov
- **Clinical Psychiatry**
  - http://www.aacap.org
  - http://www.aacp.com
  - http://www.mentalhelp.net
  - http://www.nimh.nih.gov
  - http://www.psych.org
- **Clinical Psychology**
  - http://www.aacp.com
  - http://www.apa.org

- Clinical Trials
  - http://www.centerwatch.com
  - http://www.clinicaltrials.gov
- Cloning/Human
  - http://www.ama-assn.org
  - http://www.arhp.org
  - http://www.health.nih.gov
  - http://www.humancloning.org
  - http://www.nlm.nih.gov
  - http://www.who.int
- Cold Exposure/Injury
  - http://www.ama-assn.org
  - http://www.cdc.gov/niosh
- Cold/Flu
  - http://www.aafp.org
  - http://www.cdc.gov
- Colitis
  - http://www.aafp.org
  - http://www.acg.gi.org
  - http://www.ama-assn.org
  - http://www.ccfa.org
  - http://www.niddk.nih.gov
- Colon Polyp(s)
  - http://www.acg.gi.org
  - http://www.ama-assn.org
  - http://www.fascrs.org
  - http://www.gastro.org
- Colonoscopy
  - http://www.acg.gi.org
  - http://www.gastro.org
- Colorblindness
  - http://www.aao.org
  - http://www.mcw.edu
  - http://www.nei.nih.gov
- Colorectal Cancer Screening
  - http://www.aafp.org
  - http://www.acg.gi.org
  - http://www.ama-assn.org
  - http://www.gastro.org

- Colostomy Care
  - http://www.aafp.org
  - http://www.fascrs.org
  - http://www.medhelp.org
- Coma/Stupor
  - http://www.aan.com
  - http://www.acep.com
  - http://www.acponline.org
  - http://www.ninds.nih.gov
- Communicable/Infectious Disease
  - http://www.ama-assn.org
  - http://www.aphl.org
  - http://www.cdc.gov
  - http://www.niaid.nih.gov
  - http://www.nfid.org
- Complementary/Alternative Medicine
  - http://www.ama-assn.org
  - http://www.nccam.nih.gov
  - http://www.pitt.edu~cbw.altm.html
- Concussion
  - http://www.aafp.org
  - http://www.aan.com
  - http://www.acep.com
  - http://www.biasusa.org
- Conduct Disorder
  - http://www.aap.org
  - http://www.nimh.nih.gov
  - http://www.nmha.org
- Congestive Heart Failure
  - http://www.aafp.org
  - http://www.acc.org
  - http://www.acponline.org
  - http://www.americanheart.org
  - http://www.healthcare.ucla.edu
  - http://www.nhlbi.nih.gov
- Conjunctival Hemorrhage
  - http://www.aafp.org
  - http://www.aao.org
  - http://www.nei.nih.gov

- Conjunctivitis
  - http://www.aafp.org
  - http://www.aao.org
  - http://www.nei.nih.gov
- Constipation
  - http://www.aafp.org
  - http://www.acg.gi.org
  - http://www.gastro.org
- Consumer Product Safety
  - http://www.cpsc.gov
  - http://www.fda.gov
- Contact Lens/Counseling
  - http://www.aao.org
  - http://www.cdc.gov
  - http://www.contactlenses.org
- Cor Pulmonale
  - http://www.acc.org
  - http://www.acponline.org
  - http://www.americanheart.org
  - http://www.healthcare.ucla.edu
  - http://www.nhlbi.nih.gov
- Corn/Callus/Foot
  - http://www.aafp.org
  - http://www.apma.org
- Corneal Abrasion
  - http://www.aao.org
  - http://www.nei.nih.gov
  - http://www.preventblindness.org
- Corneal Transplant/Eye
  - http://www.aao.org
  - http://www.nei.nih.gov
- Coronary Artery Bypass
  - http://www.acc.org
  - http://www.nhlbi.nih.gov
  - http://www.sts.org
- Cosmetic Surgery
  - http://www.plasticsurgery.org
  - http://www.yoursurgery.com

- Costochrondritis/Tietze's Syndrome
  - http://www.aafp.org
  - http://www.arthritis.org
  - http://www.chestnet.org
- Cough
  - http://www.aafp.org
  - http://www.chestnet.org
  - http://www.lungusa.org
- Critical Care Medicine
  - http://www.acep.com
  - http://www.sccm.org
- Crohn's Disease
  - http://www.acg.gi.org
  - http://www.acponline.org
  - http://www.ccfa.org
  - http://www.gastro.org
- Croup
  - http://www.aafp.org
  - http://www.aap.org
  - http://www.kidshealth.org
- Crutzfeldt-Jacob Disease/Variant
  - http://www.aan.com
  - http://www.healthsystem.virginia.edu
  - http://www.ninds.nih.gov
  - http://www.who.int
- Cystic Fibrosis
  - http://www.aafp.org
  - http://www.aap.org
  - http://www.cff.org
- Cystitis
  - http://www.aafp.org
  - http://www.afud.org
  - http://www.auanet.org
  - http://www.ichelp.org
  - http://www.niddk.nih.gov
- Cystocele
  - http://www.aafp.org
  - http://www.acog.org
  - http://www.auanet.org

- http://www.ichelp.org
- http://www.niddk.nih.gov

2.4   Deafness to Dysuria

- Deafness
  - http://www.entnet.org
  - http://www.nidcd.nih.gov
  - http://www.mc.vanderbilt.edu
- Death and Dying
  - http://www.death_dying.org
  - http://www.hospicenet.org
- Deep Venous Thrombosis/Leg(s)
  - http://www.aafp.org
  - http://www.acponline.org
- Dehydration
  - http;//www.aafp.org
  - http://www.acponline.org
- Delirium
  - http://www.aafp.org
  - http://www.aan.com
  - http://www.acponline.org
  - http://www.ninds.nih.gov
- Dementia/Organic Brain Syndrome
  - http://www.aafp.org
  - http://www.aan.com
  - http://www.americangeriatrics.org
  - http://www.nia.nih.gov
  - http://www.ninds.nih.gov
- Dental Disease
  - http://www.ada.org
  - http://www.hsdm.med.harvard.edu
  - http://www.perio.org
- Depression/Bipolar
  - http://www.aafp.org
  - http://www.mentalhelp.net
  - http://www.nimh.nih.gov.
  - http://www.nmha.org
  - http://www.psych.org

- **Depression/Dysthymia**
  - http://www.aafp.org
  - http://www.mentalhelp.net
  - http://www.nimh.nih.gov
  - http://www.nmha.org
  - http://www.psych.org
- **Depression/Major**
  - http://www.aafp.org
  - http://www.mentalhelp.net
  - http://www.nimh.nih.gov
  - http://www.nmha.org
  - http://www.psych.org
- **Dermabrasion**
  - http://www.aad.org
  - http://www.asds-net.org
- **Dermatitis/Contact**
  - http://www.aad.org
  - http://www.aafp.org
- **Dermatologic Surgery**
  - http://www.asds-net.org
  - http://www.mohscollege.org
- **Dermatomyositits**
  - http://www.aarda.org
  - http://www.acponline.org
  - http://www.medhelp.org
  - http://www.myositis.org
- **Diabetes Mellitus**
  - http://www.aafp.org
  - http://www.acponline.org
  - http://www.cdc.gov/diabetes
  - http://www.diabetes.org
  - http://www.endo-society.org
  - http://www.jdrf.org
  - http://www.niddk.nih.gov
- **Diabetes Mellitus/Foot Care**
  - http://www.aafp.org
  - http://www.acponline.org
  - http://www.aofas.org
  - http://www.apma.org

- Diaper Rash
  - http://www.aad.org
  - http://www.aafp.org
  - http://www.aap.org
- Diaphoresis/Sweating
  - http:www.aad.org
  - http://www.aafp.org
  - http://www.acponline.org
  - http://www.medhelp.org
  - http://www.sweathelp.org
- Diarrhea/Dehydration
  - http://www.aafp.org
  - http://www.aap.org
  - http://www.acg.gi.org
- Dietary Guidelines
  - http://www.ama-assn.org
  - http://www.americanheart.org
  - http://www.health.gov/dietaryguidelines
  - http://www.usda.gov
- Dietary Supplements
  - http://www.ama-assn.org
  - http://www.fda.gov
  - http://www.nal.usda.gov
  - http://www.od.nih.gov
- Dieting
  - http://www.aafp.org
  - http://www.ama-assn.org
  - http://www.cyberdiet.com
  - http://www.eatright.org
- Digestive Disease/Health
  - http://www.aafp.org
  - http://www.acg.gi.org
  - http://www.asge.org
  - http://www.ccfa.org
  - http://www.fdhn.org
  - http://www.gastro.org
  - http://www.iffgd.org
  - http://www.niddk.nih.gov

- **Disability Evaluation/Physicians**
  - http://www.aadep.org
  - http://www.ama-assn.org
- **Disease Prevention**
  - http://www.acpm.org
  - http://www.cdc.gov
  - http://www.od.nih.gov
- **Dislocation/Shoulder**
  - http://www.aafp.org
  - http;//www.aaos.org
  - http://www.niams.nih.gov
- **Diverticulitis/Colon**
  - http://www.aafp.org
  - http://www.acg.gi.org
  - http://www.fascrs.org
  - http;//www.gastro.org
- **Dizziness/Vertigo**
  - http://www.aafp.org
  - http://www.acponline.org
  - http://www.aan.com
- **Down's Syndrome**
  - http://www.aap.org
  - http://www.nads.org
  - http://www.ndss.org
  - http://www.nlm.nih.gov
- **Drowning/Nonfatal**
  - http://www.aafp.org
  - http://www.acep.com
  - http://www.cpsc.gov
- **Drug Abuse**
  - http://www.aap.org
  - http://www.niaaa.nih.gov
  - http://www.nida.nih.gov
  - http://www.nmha.org
- **Dry Eye Syndrome**
  - http://www.aafp.org
  - http://www.aao.org
  - http://www.nei.nih.gov
  - http://www.preventblindness.org

- Dupuytren's Contracture
  - http://www.aafp.org
  - http://www.aaos.org
  - http://www.healthcare.ucla.edu
  - http;//www.healthsystem.virginia.edu
- Dwarfism
  - http://www.aafp.org
  - http://www.aap.org
  - http://www.healthcare.ucla.edu
  - http://www.nichd.nih.gov
- Dysarthria/Stroke Speech Defect
  - http://www.nidcd.nih.gov
  - http://www.ninds.nih.gov
  - http://www.stroke.org
- Dysgeusia/Taste Disorder
  - http://www.aafp.org
  - http://www.medhelp.org
  - http://www.ninds.nih.gov
- Dyslexia/Learning Disorder
  - http://www.healthcare.ucla.edu
  - http://www.healthsystem.virginia.edu
  - http://www.kidshealth.org
  - http://www.nidcd.nih.gov
- Dysmenorrhea/Painful Menstruation
  - http://www.aafp.org
  - http://www.acog.org
  - http://www.fda.gov
- Dyspareunia/Painful Intercourse
  - http://www.aafp.org
  - http://www.acog.org
  - http://www.ichelp.org
- Dyspepsia/Heartburn
  - http://www.aafp.org
  - http://www.gastro.org
  - http://www.niddk.nih.gov
- Dysphagia/Difficulty Swallowing
  - http://www.aafp.org
  - http://www.acg.gi.org
  - http://www.acponline.org
  - http://www.gastro.org

- Dysplastic Nevi/Skin Moles
  - http://www.aad.org
  - http://www.aafp.org
  - http://www.cancer.gov
- Dyspnea/Shortness of Breath
  - http://www.aafp.org
  - http://www.acc.org
  - http://www.acponline.org
- Dysuria/Painful Urination
  - http://www.aafp.org
  - http://www.auanet.org
  - http://www.niddk.nih.gov

2.5   Ear/Nose/Throat Diseases to Eye Injury

- Ear Nose Throat Diseases
  - http://www.aafp.org
  - http://www.aaoaf.org
  - http://www.allergy-ent.org
  - http://www.entnet.org
- Earwax/Impacted
  - http://www.aafp.org
  - http://www.audiology.org
  - http://www.entent.org
- Eating Disorders
  - http://www.aafp.org
  - http://www.ama-assn.org
  - http://www.anad.org
  - http://www.eatingdorders.org
  - http://www.mentalhelp.net
  - http://www.nimh.nih.gov
  - http://www.nmha.org
  - http://www.psych.org
- Ebola Virus
  - http://www.cdc.gov
  - http://www.niaid.nih.gov
- Eczema/Atopic Dermatatitis
  - http://www.aad.org

- http://www.aafp.org
- http://www.niams.nih.gov

- **Edema/Leg(s)**
  - http://www.aafp.org
  - http://www.acc.org
  - http://www.acponline.org

- **Elder Abuse**
  - http://www.aafp.org
  - http://www.cdc.gov
  - http://www.elderabusecenter.org
  - http://www.webmd.com

- **Electric Current Injury**
  - http://www.acep.com
  - http://www.cdc.gov/niosh

- **Emphysema**
  - http://www.aafp.org
  - http://www.acponline.org
  - http://www.chestnet.org
  - http://www.lungusa.org
  - http://www.nhlbi.nih.gov
  - http://www.sts.org

- **Encephalitis**
  - http://www.aafp.org
  - http://www.aan.com
  - http://www.niaid.nih.gov
  - http://www.webmd.com

- **Endocrine Disorders**
  - http://www.aace.com/college
  - http://www.diabetes.org
  - http://www.endo-society.org
  - http://www.tsh.org

- **Endometriosis**
  - http://www.aafp.org
  - http://www.acog.org
  - http://www.4women
  - http://www.healthywomen.org

- **Enuresis/Bed Wetting**
  - http://www.aafp.org
  - http://www.aap.org

- **Environmental Disease/Health**
  - http://www.acoem.org
  - http://www.aiha.org
  - http://www.aphl.org
  - http://www.cdc.gov/ncipc
  - http://www.cdc.gov/niosh
  - http://www.niehs.nih.gov
  - http://www.osha.gov
- **Epidemic Disease**
  - http://www.acpm.org
  - http://www.ama-assn.org
  - http://www.cdc.gov
- **Epididymitis/Testicular Disorder**
  - http://www.aafp.org
  - http://www.auanet.org
- **Epiglottitis**
  - http://www.aafp.org
  - http://www.aap.org
  - http://www.acponline.org
- **Epilepsy**
  - http://www.aesnet.org
  - http://www.epilepsyfoundation.org
  - http://www.ninds.nih.gov
- **Epistaxes/Nose Bleeding**
  - http://www.aafp.org
  - http://www.acponline.org
  - http://www.entnet.org
- **Esophagitis/Barrett's**
  - http://www.acg.gi.org
  - http://www.gastro.org
  - http://www.healthsystem.virginia.edu
  - http://www.niddk.nih.gov
- **Eustacian Tube Dysfunction**
  - http://www.aao.org
  - http://www.aaoaf.org
  - http://www.entnet.org
- **Exhaustion/Exposure**
  - http://www.aafp.org
  - http://www.acep.org
  - http://www.cdc.gov/niosh

- Eye Disorders
  - http://www.aao.org
  - http://www.afb.org
  - http://www.eyenet.org
  - http://www.glaucoma.org
  - http://www.isrs.org
  - http://www.lighthouse.org
  - http://www.nei.nih.gov
  - http://www.preventblindness.org
- Eye Exam/Preventive/Adults
  - http://www.aao.org
  - http://www.ama-assn.org
  - http://www.glaucoma.org
  - http://www.preventblindness.org
- Eye Glass Safety/Counseling
  - http://www.aao.org
  - http://www.nei.nih.gov
  - http://www.preventblindness.org
- Eye Injury
  - http://www.aao.org
  - http://www.cdc.gov/niosh
  - http://www.eyenet.org
  - http://www.nei.nih.gov
  - http://www.preventblindness.org

2.6 Facial Pain to Fractures

- Facial Pain
  - http://www.aafp.org
  - http://www.aahcfp.org
  - http://www.entnet.org
  - http://www.medhelp.org
- Facial Skin Rejuvenation
  - http://www.aad.org
  - http://www.asds-net.org
  - http://www.facial-plastic-surgery.org
- Family Medicine
  - http://www.aafp.org
  - http://www.ama-assn.org

- Fatigue
  - http://www.aafp.org
  - http://www.acponline.org
  - http://www.clevelandclinic.org
  - http://www.healthsystem.virginia.edu
  - http://www.medhelp.org
- Febrile Seizure
  - http://www.aafp.org
  - http://www.aap.org
  - http://www.acponline.org
  - http://www.ninds.nih.gov
- Fetal Alcohol Syndrome
  - http://www.aafp.org
  - http://www.aap.org
  - http://www.acog.org
- Fever
  - http://www.aafp.org
  - http://www.acponline.org
- Fibromyalgia
  - http://www.aafp.org
  - http://www.arthritis.org
  - http://www.cfidsfoundation.org
  - http://www.rheumatology.org
- First Aid
  - http://www.aafp.org
  - http://www.ama-assn.org
  - http://www.cdc.gov
  - http://www.webmd.com
- Flatulence/Gas
  - http://www.aafp.org
  - http://www.acg.gi.org
  - http://www.gastro.org
- Floaters/Vitreous/Eye
  - http://www.aao.org
  - http://www.eyenet.org
  - http://www.nei.nih.gov
  - http://www.preventblindness.org
- Food Allergy/Anaphylaxis
  - http://www.cfsan.fda.gov

- http://www.foodallergy.org
- http://www.foodsafety.gov
- Foodborne Diseases
  - http://www.ama-assn.org
  - http://www.aphl.org
  - http://www.cdc.gov
  - http://www.fda.gov
  - http://www.foodsafety.gov
  - http://www.usda.gov/cnpp
  - http://www.who.int
- Foot/Ankle Disorders/Injury
  - http://www.aofas.org
  - http://www.apma.org
- Fractures
  - http://www.aafp.org
  - http://www.aanos.org
  - http://www.aaos.org
  - http://www.acsm.org

2.7   Gallbladder Disease to Gynecological Exam

- Gallbladder Disease/Gallstones
  - http://www.aafp.org
  - http://www.acg.gi.org
  - http://www.gastro.org
  - http://www.niddk.nih.gov
- Gambling Addiction
  - http://www.gamblersanonymous.org
  - http://www.ncpgambling.org
- Ganglion Cyst
  - http://www.aafp.org
  - http://www.aaos.org
- Gastroenteritis
  - http://www.aafp.org
  - http://www.acg.gi.org
  - http://www.gastro.org
  - http://www.niddk.nih.gov

- **Gastro-Esophogeal Reflux Disease/GERD**
  - http://www.aafp.org
  - http://www.acg.gi.org
  - http://www.gastro.org
  - http://www.niddk.nih.gov
- **Gastrointestinal Disease**
  - http://www.acg.gi.org
  - http://www.gastro.org
  - http://www.medhelp.org
  - http://www.niddk.nih.gov
- **Gastrointestinal Disorders/Functional**
  - http://www.gastro.org
  - http://www.iffgd.org
  - http://www.niddk.nih.gov
- **Gastrointestinal Endoscopy/Upper GI**
  - http://www.acg.go.org
  - http://www.gastro.org
  - http://www.sages.org
- **Genetic Disorders/Counseling**
  - http://www.aap.org
  - http://www.acmg.net
  - http://www.nhgri.nih.gov
- **Genital Warts**
  - http://www.aafp.org
  - http://www.acponline.org
  - http://www.ashastd.org
  - http://www.cdc.gov
- **Geriatric Medicine**
  - http://www.aafp.org
  - http://www.americangeriatrics.org
  - http://www.nia.nih.gov
- **Giardiasis**
  - http://www.aafp.org
  - http://www.acponline.org
  - http://www.cdc.gov
- **Glaucoma**
  - http://www.aafp.org
  - http://www.glaucoma.org
  - http://www.nei.nih.gov

- Glomerulonephritis
  - http://www.aafp.org
  - http://www.acponline.org
  - http://www.kidney.org
  - http://www.niddk.nih.gov
- Glycosuria
  - http://www.aafp.org
  - http://www.acponline.org
  - http://www.diabetes.org
- Goiter
  - http://www.aafp.org
  - http://www.acponline.org
  - http://www.the-thyroid-society.org
  - http://www.tsh.org
- Gout
  - http://www.aafp.org
  - http://www.acponline.org
  - http://www.arthritis.org
- Guillain-Barre Syndrome
  - http://www.aafp.org
  - http://www.aan.com
  - http://www.healthsystem.virginia.edu
  - http://www.ninds.nih.gov
- Gum/Periodontal Disease
  - http://www.ada.org
  - http://www.noah-health.org
  - http://www.perio.org
- Gynecological Exam
  - http://www.acog.org
  - http://www.healthywomen.org
  - http://www.womenshealthmatters.ca

2.8 Hair Pulling to Hypothyroidism

- Hair Pulling/Trichotillomania
  - http://www.aad.org
  - http://www.aafp.org
  - http://www.mayoclinic.com

- http://www.psych.org
- http://www.trich.org
- Hair Restoration
  - http://www.asds-net.org
  - http://www.clevelandclinic.org
- Halitosis
  - http://www.aafp.org
  - http://www.ada.org
  - http://www.webmd.com
- Hammertoe
  - http://www.apma.org
  - http://www.aofas.org
- Hand/Surgery
  - http://www.assh.org
  - http://www.hand_surgery.org
- Hangover
  - http://www.aafp.org
  - http://www.ama-assn.org
  - http://www.mayoclinic.com
  - http://www.webmd.com
- Headache
  - http://www.aafp.org
  - http://www.aahcfp.org
  - http://www.achenet.org
  - http://www.ahsnet.org
  - http://www.headaches.org
- Head Injury
  - http://www.aan.com
  - http://www.aans.org
  - http://www.acep.com
  - http://www.biausa.org
- Head/Neck/Facial Pain
  - http://www.aahcfp.org
  - http://www.ampainsoc.org
  - http://www.clevelandclinic.org
- Healthcare Quality
  - http://www.ahrq.gov
  - http://www.ama-assn.org
  - http://www.guideline.gov

- http://www.hon.ch
- http://www.who.int
- Health Checkup/Adults
  - http://www.aafp.org
  - http://www.acponline.org
  - http://www.ahrq.gov
  - http://www.ama-assn.org
  - http://www.clevelandclinic.org
  - http://www.healthfinder.gov
- Healthfinder Organizations Directory
  - http://www.ama-assn.org
  - http://www.healthfinder.org
- Health Information
  - http://www.ama-assn.org
  - http://www.health.nih.gov
  - http://www.intellihealth.com
  - http://www.iom.edu
- Health Insurance/Medicare/VA
  - http://www.ama-assn.org
  - http://www.healthfinder.gov
  - http://www.medicare.gov
  - http://www1.va.gov/health_benefits
- Health Quackery/Elderly
  - http://www.ama-assn.org
  - http://www.americangeriatrics.org
  - http://www.healthsystem.virginia.edu
  - http://www.nia.nih.gov
- Healthy Lifestyle
  - http://www.aafp.org
  - http://www.acpm.org
  - http://www.ama-assn.org
  - http://www.cdc.gov
  - http://www.healthypeople.gov
  - http://www.noah-health.org
- Healthy People 2010
  - http://www.healthypeople.gov
- Hearing Aid/Counseling
  - http://www.audiology.org
  - http://www.entnet.org
  - http://www.nia.nih.gov

- **Hearing Disorders/Loss**
  - http://www.aafp.org
  - http://www.allergy_ent.org
  - http://www.audiology.org
  - http://www.entnet.org
  - http://www.nia.nih.gov
  - http://www.nidcd.nih.gov
- **Heart Block**
  - http://www.aafp.org
  - http://www.acc.org
  - http://www.americanheart.org
  - http://www.nhlbi.nih.gov
- **Heartburn**
  - http://www.aafp.org
  - http://www.acg.gi.org
  - http://www.gastro.org
- **Heart Disease**
  - http://www.aafp.org
  - http://www.acc.org
  - http://www.americanheart.org
  - http://www.nhlbi.nih.gov
- **Heart/Lung Transplantation**
  - http://www.ishlt.org
  - http://www.clevelandclinic.org
  - http://www.healthsystem.virginia.edu
  - http://www.nhlbi.nih.gov
- **Heart Surgery**
  - http://www.clevelandclinic.org
  - http://www.healthcare.ucla.edu
  - http://www.nhlbi.nih.gov
  - http://www.sts.org
  - http://www.yoursurgery.com
- **Heat Injury/Sunburn**
  - http://www.aad.org
  - http://www.aafp.org
  - http://www.acponline.org
  - http://www.cdc.gov/niosh
- **Hemachromatosis**
  - http://www.aafp.org

- http://www.acponline.org
- http://www.clevelandclinic.org
- http://www.irondisorders.org
- http://www.liverfoundation.org
- http://www.medhelp.org
- Hemangioma/Skin
  - http://www.aad.org
  - http://www.aafp.org
  - http://www.aap.org
- Hematuria/Blood in Urine
  - http://www.aafp.org
  - http://www.auanet.org
  - http://www.kidney.org
  - http://www.niddk.nih.gov
- Hemorrhagic Fever
  - http://www.acponline.org
  - http://www.cdc.gov
  - http://www.healthcare.ucla.edu
  - http://www.niaid.nih.gov
- Hemorrhoids
  - http://www.aafp.org
  - http://www.facrs.org
- Hepatitis
  - http://www.acponline.org
  - http://www.cdc.gov
  - http://www.hepfi.org
  - http://www.liverfoundation.org
- Herbal Supplements
  - http://www.ama-assn.org
  - http://www.fda.gov
  - http://www.herbalgram.org
  - http://www.nal.usda.gov
  - http://www.nccam.nih.gov
  - http://www.ods.od.nih.gov
- Herberden's Nodes
  - http://www.aafp.org
  - http;//www.aaos.org
- Hermaphroditism
  - http://www.aap.org

- http://www.healthcare.ucla.edu
- http://www.nacd.org
- Hernia
  - http://www.aafp.org
  - http://www.acg.gi.org
  - http://www.facs.org
  - http://www.niddk.nih.gov
  - http://www.yoursurgery.com
- Herpes/Genital
  - http://www.aafp.org
  - http://www.acog.org
  - http://www.acponline.org
  - http://www.ashastd.org
  - http://www.cdc.gov
- Herpes/Simplex
  - http://www.aafp.org
  - http://www.acponline.org
  - http://www.niaid.nih.gov
  - http://www.nfid.nih.gov
- Herpes Zoster/Shingles
  - http://www.aafp.org
  - http://www.acponline.org
  - http;//www.health.nih.gov
  - http://www.medhelp.org
  - http://www.niaid.nih.gov
- Hip Disorders
  - http://www.aaos.org
  - http://www.arthritis.org
  - http://www.niams.nih.gov
  - http://www.rheumatology.org
- Hirsutism
  - http://www.aace.com/college
  - http://www.aafp.org
  - http://www.medhelp.org
- Home Health Care
  - http://www.aafp.org
  - http://www.aahsa.org
  - http://www.ama-assn.org
  - http://www.nahc.org

- **Hormone Replacement Therapy**
  - http://www.aafp.org
  - http://www.acog.org
  - http://www.ama-assn.org
  - http://www.cdc.gov
  - http://www.4women.gov
  - http://www.womenshealthmatters.ca
- **Hospice/Palliative Medicine**
  - http://www.aahpm.org
  - http://www.hospicenet.org
- **Hospital Directory/International**
  - http://www.bowyer.org.uk/hospital.htm
- **Hospital Directory/USA**
  - http://www.healthfinder.gov
- **Huntington's Disease**
  - http://www.aan.com
  - http://www.healthcare.ucla.edu
  - http://www.healthsystem.virginia.edu
  - http://www.ninds.nih.gov
- **Hydrocephalous**
  - http://www.aans.org
  - http://www.aap.org
  - http://www.healthcare.ucla.edu
  - http://www.healthsystem.virginia.edu
  - http://www.ninds.nih.gov
- **Hyperlipidemia/Hypercholesterolemia**
  - http://www.acc.org
  - http://www.acponline.org
  - http://www.americanheart.org
  - http://www.nhlbi.nih.gov
- **Hypertension/Elevated Blood Pressure**
  - http://www.acc.org
  - http://www.acponline.org
  - http://www.americanheart.org
  - http://www.nhlbi.nih.gov
- **Hyperthyroidism**
  - http://www.aafp.org
  - http://www.acponline.org

- http://www.the-thyroid-society.org
- http://www.tsh.org
- Hypnosis
  - http://www.ama-assn.org
  - http://www.apa.org
  - http://www.nimh.nih.gov
  - http://www.psych.org
- Hypothermia
  - http://www.aafp.org
  - http://www.aap.org
  - http://www.acep.org
  - http://www.americangeriatrics.org
  - http://www.nia.nih.gov
- Hypothyroidism
  - http://www.aafp.org
  - http://www.acponline.org
  - http://www.the-thyroid-society.org
  - http://www.tsh.org

2.9   Immunizations to Irritable Bowel

- Immunizations/Schedules
  - http://www.aafp.org
  - http://www.acpm.org
  - http://www.ama-assn.org
  - http://www.aphl.org
  - http://www.cdc.gov
  - http://www.tripprep.com
- Immunological Disorders
  - http://www.aaaai.org
  - http://www.aai.org
  - http://www.aarda.org
  - http://www.healthcare.ucla.edu
  - http://www.healthsystem.virginia.edu
- Impetigo
  - http://www.aad.org
  - http://www.aafp.org

- Impotence
  - http://www.aafp.org
  - http://www.auanet.org
  - http://www.clevelandclinic.org
  - http://www.ivf.org
  - http://www.maleinfertility.org
  - http://www.niddk.nih.gov
- Incontinence/Urinary/Bowel
  - http://www.aafp.org
  - http://www.acg.gi.org
  - http://www.afud.org
  - http://www.auanet.org
  - http://www.fascrs.org
  - http://www.nafc.org
- Infectious Disease
  - http://www.cdc.gov
  - http://www.nfid.org
  - http://www.niaid.nih.gov
- Infectious Mononucleosis
  - http://www.aafp.org
  - http://www.aap.org
  - http://www.niaid.nih.gov
- Infertility
  - http://www.asrm.org
  - http://www.ivf.org
  - http://www.maleinfertility.org
  - http://www.medhelp.org
- Influenza/Vaccination
  - http://www.aafp.org
  - http://www.ama-assn.org
  - http://www.cdc.gov
  - http://www.who.int
- Ingrown Toenail
  - http://www.aafp.org
  - http://www.apma.gov
- Inhalant Abuse
  - http://www.aap.org
  - http://www.kidshealth.org
  - http://www.nida.nih.gov

- **Injury Prevention**
  - http://www.aafp.org
  - http://www.aaos.org
  - http://www.aapmr.org
  - http://www.acpm.org
  - http://www.acsm.org
  - http://www.cdc.gov/ncipc
- **Insect Bite/Non-Venomous**
  - http://www.aafp.org
  - http://www.cdc.gov/noish
- **Internal Medicine**
  - http://www.acponline.org
  - http://www.asim.org
  - http://www.sgim.org
- **Intestinal Obstruction**
  - http://www.aafp.org
  - http://www.acg.gi.org
  - http://www.gastro.org
  - http://www.niddk.nih.gov
- **Irritable Bowel Syndrome**
  - http;//www.aafp.org
  - http://www.acg.gi.org
  - http://www.acponline.org
  - http://www.gastro.org
  - http://www.iffgd.org

2.10 Joint Disease to Joint Replacement

- **Joint Disease**
  - http://www.acsm.org
  - http://www.arthritis.org
  - http://www.niams.nih.gov
  - http://www.rheumatology.org
- **Joint Replacement**
  - http://www.aaos.org
  - http://www.arthritis.org
  - http://www.clevelandclinic.org

2.11 Kawasaki Disease to Knee Disorders

- Kawasaki Disease
  - http://www.aafp.org
  - http://www.aap.org
  - http://www.medhelp.org
- Kidney Disease/Cyst
  - http://www.aafp.org
  - http://www.acponline
  - http://www.auanet.org
  - http://www.kidney.org
  - http://www.niddk.nih.gov
- Kleinfelter's Syndrome
  - http://www.aace.com/college
  - http://www.aap.org
  - http://www.acmg.net
- Knee Disorders
  - http://www.aafp.org
  - http://www.aap.org
  - http://www.aaos.org
  - http://www.arthritis.org
  - http://www.niams.nih.gov

2.12 Lab Tests to Lymphoma

- Lab Tests/Abnormalities
  - http://www.labtestsonline.org
- Lactose Intolerance
  - http://www.acg.gi.org
  - http://www.gastro.org
  - http://www.medhelp.org
- Laparoscopic Surgery
  - http://www.facs.org
  - http://www.clevelandclinic.org
  - http://www.sages.org
  - http://www.yoursurgery.com

- Laryngitis
  - http://www.aafp.org
  - http://www.aap.org
  - http://www.webmd.com
- Learning Disabilities
  - http://www.aap.org
  - http://www.healthcare.ucla.edu
  - http://www.ldanatl.org
  - http://www.kidshealth.org
  - http://www.nichd.nih.gov
- Leprosy
  - http://www.cdc.gov
  - http://www.medhelp.org
  - http://www.niaid.nih.gov
- Leukemia
  - http://www.cancer.gov
  - http://www.clevelandclinic.org
  - http://www.healthcare.ucla.edu
  - http://www.leukemia.org
- Lice
  - http://www.aafp.org
  - http://www.aap.org
  - http://www.kidshealth.org
- Lifting Safety
  - http://www.aafp.org
  - http://www.aaos.org
  - http://www.acpm.org
  - http://www.cdc.gov
- Lipoma
  - http://www.aad.org
  - http://www.cancer.gov
  - http;//www.medhelp.org
- Liposuction
  - http://www.asds-net.org
  - http://www.clevelandclinic.org
  - http://www.facs.org
  - http;//www.medhelp.org
  - http://www.yoursurgery.com
  - http://www.webmd.com

- Liver Disease
  - http://www.aafp.org
  - http://www.acponline.org
  - http://www.gastro.org
  - http://www.hepfi.org
  - http://www.liverfoundation.org
  - http://www.niddk.nih.gov
- Liver Transplantation
  - http://www.liverfoundation.org
  - http://www.niddk.nih.gov
- Long Term Care
  - http://www.aafp.org
  - http://www.ama-assn-org
  - http://www.americangeriatrics.org
  - http://www.geron.org
  - http://www.nahc.org
- Lumbar Disk Disease/Low Back Pain
  - http://www.aafp.org
  - http://www.aans.org
  - http://www.aaos.org
- Lung Disease
  - http://www.chestnet.org
  - http://www.lungusa.org
  - http://www.nhlbi.nih.gov
- Lupus
  - http://www.aarda.org
  - http://www.acponline.org
  - http://www.healthcare.ucla.edu
  - http://www.healthsystem.virginia.edu
  - http://www.lupus.org
- Lyme Disease
  - http://www.aafp.org
  - http://www.acponline.org
  - http://www.cdc.gov
  - http://www.niaid.nih.gov
- Lymphatic Disorders
  - http://www.heathcare.ucla.edu
  - http://www.healthsystem.virginia.edu
  - http://www.nhlbi.nih.gov

- Lymphedema
  - http://www.komen.org
  - http://www.lymphnet.org
  - http://www.oncolink.upenn.edu
- Lymphoma/Hodgkins/Non-Hodgkins
  - http://www.acponline.org
  - http://www.cancer.gov
  - http://www.medhelp.org

2.13 Macular Degeneration to Myopathy/Muscle Wasting

- Macular Degeneration
  - http://www.aafp.org
  - http://www.aao.org
  - http://www.nei.nih.gov
  - http://www.preventblindness.org
- Mad Cow Disease
  - http://www.aan.com
  - http://www.ninds.nih.gov
  - http://www.who.int
- Malaria
  - http://www.aafp.org
  - http://www.acponline.org
  - http://www.aphl.org
  - http://www.cdc.gov
  - http://www.niaid.nih.gov
  - http://www.who.int
- Male Genitourinary Disease
  - http://www.aafp.org
  - http://www.afud.org
  - http://www.cdc.gov
  - http://www.niddk.nih.gov
- Mammography
  - http://www.cancer.gov
  - http://www.4women.org
  - http://www.womenshealthmatters.ca

- Manipulation/Osteopathic
  - http://www.aoa-net.org
  - http://www.aoa-net.org/Consumers/consumers.htm
  - http://www.osteopathic.org
- Marijuana Use/Abuse
  - http://www.aafp.org
  - http://www.aap.org
  - http://www.kidshealth.org
  - http://www.nida.nih.gov
- Measles
  - http://www.aafp.org
  - http://www.aap.org
  - http://www.kidshealth.org
- Medical College/School Directory/USA & International
  - http://www.aamc.org
  - http://www.bowyer.org.uk/med_sch.htm
- Medical Dictionary/Encyclopedia
  - http://www.ama-assn.org
  - http://www.healthfinder.gov
  - http://www.medlineplus.gov
- Medical Errors
  - http://www.ahrq.gov
  - http://www.ahrq.gov/consumer/20tips.htm
  - http://www.ahrq.gov/qual/errors.htm
  - http://www.cdc.gov
  - http://www.medhelp.org
  - http://www.who.int
- Medical Ethics
  - http://www.ama-assn.org
  - http://www.who.int
- Medication Counseling/Elderly
  - http://www.americangeriatrics.org
  - http://www.nia.nih.gov
- Meditation
  - http://www.mbmi.org
  - http://www.netwellness.org
  - http://www.umassmed.edu.cfm
  - http://www.webmd.com
  - http://www.wellness-community.org

- **Melanoma/Malignant**
  - http://www.aad.org
  - http://www.healthcare.ucla.edu
  - http://www.healthsystem.virginia.edu
  - http://www.cancer.gov
- **Memory Loss/Elderly**
  - http://www.aafp.org
  - http://www.americangeriatrics.org
  - http://www.aoa.dhhs.gov
  - http://www.nia.nih.gov
- **Meneire's Disease**
  - http://www.aafp.org
  - http://www.aao.org
  - http://www.hon.ch
  - http://www.nidcd.nih.gov
- **Meningitis**
  - http://www.aafp.org
  - http://www.aan.org
  - http://www.acponline.org
  - http://www.cdc.gov
  - http://www.ninds.nih.gov
- **Menopause**
  - http://www.aafp.org
  - http://www.acog.org
  - http://www.menopause.org
  - http://www.womenshealthmatters.ca
- **Men's Health**
  - http://www.aafp.org
  - http://www.ama-assn.org
  - http://www.intellihealth.com
  - http://www.mayoclinic.com
  - http://www.noah-health.org
  - http://www.webmd.com
- **Mental Health/Disorders**
  - http://www.aacap.org
  - http://www.aacp.com
  - http://www.apa.org
  - http://www.cyberpsych.org
  - http://www.helping.apa.org

- http://www.mentalhelp.net
- http://www.nami.org
- http://www.nida.nih.gov
- http://www.nimh.nih.gov
- http://www.nmha.org
- http://www.psych.org
- http://www.psychosomatic.org
- http://www.who.int
- Mental Retardation
  - http://www.aacap.org
  - http://www.aamr.org
  - http://www.aap.org
  - http://www.nads.org
  - http://www.ndss.org
  - http://www.nichd.gov
  - http://www.nmha.org
  - http://www.thearc.org
- Mindfullness
  - http://www.mbmi.org
  - http://www.umassmed.edu/cfm
- Mitral Value Prolapse
  - http://www.aafp.org
  - http://www.acc.org
  - http://www.acponline.org
  - http://www.americanheart.org
- Mohs Micrographic Skin Surgery
  - http://www.mohscollege.org
  - http://www.skincancerinfo.com
- Molluscum Conagiosum
  - http://www.acponline.org
  - http://www.ashastd.org
  - http://www.clevelandclinic.org
  - http://www.healthcare.ucla.edu
  - http://www.medhelp.org
- Mosquito Borne Diseases
  - http://www.aafp.org
  - http://www.acponline.org
  - http://www.cdc.gov

- **Mouth Disease**
  - http://www.aafp.org
  - http://www.ada.org
  - http://www.webmd.com
- **Mouth/Teeth Care/Elderly**
  - http://www.aafp.org
  - http://www.ada.org
  - http://www.hsdm.med.harvard.edu
  - http://www.nia.nih.gov
- **Movement Disorder**
  - http://www.aan.com
  - http://www.medhelp.org
  - http://www.ninds.nih.gov
  - http://www.wemove.org
- **Multiple Myeloma**
  - http://www.cancer.gov
  - http://www.clevelandclinic.org
  - http://www.healthsystem.virginia.edu
- **Multiple Sclerosis**
  - http://www.acponline.org
  - http://www.healthcare.ucla.edu
  - http://www.msif.org/en
  - http://www.ninds.nih.gov
  - http://www.nmss.org
- **Mumps**
  - http://www.aafp.org
  - http://www.aap.org
  - http://www.cdc.gov
  - http://www.kidshealth.org
- **Muscle Cramps**
  - http://www.aafp.org
  - http://www.acponline.org
  - http://www.webmd.com
- **Muscular Dystropy**
  - http://www.healthcare.ucla.edu
  - http://www.mdausa.org
  - http://www.webmd.com

- **Musculoskeletal Disorders**
  - http://www.aaos.org
  - http://www.aofas.org
  - http://www.apma.org
  - http://www.backpainreliefonline.com
  - http://www.cfidsfoundation.org
  - http://www.mdausa.org
  - http://www.myositis.org
  - http://www.niams.nih.gov
  - http://www.nof.org
  - http://www.spine_health.com
  - http://www.wemove.org
- **Myasthenia gravis**
  - http://www.aarda.org
  - http://www.clevelandclinic.org
  - http://www.healthcare.edu
  - http://www.niams.nih.gov
- **Myocardial Infarction**
  - http://www.acc.org
  - http://www.acponline.org
  - http://www.americanheart.org
  - http://www.nhlbi.nih.gov
- **Myoclonus**
  - http://www.aafp.org
  - http://www.aan.com
  - http://www.acponline.org
  - http://www.healthcare.ucla.edu
  - http://www.medhelp.org
  - http://www.ninds.nih.gov
- **Myopathy/Muscle Wasting**
  - http://www.aafp.org
  - http://www.mayoclinic.com
  - http://www.myositis.org
  - http://www.niams.nih.gov
  - http://www.rheumatology.org

2.14 Nail Disease to Nutrition

- Nail Disease/Fingers
  - http://www.aad.org
  - http://www.aafp.org
- Nail Disease/Toenails
  - http://www.aafp.org
  - http://www.apma.org
- Narcolepsy
  - http://www.aafp.org
  - http://www.clevelandclinic.org
  - http://www.nhlbi.nih.gov
  - http://www.sleepfoundation.org
- National Senior Citizen Law Center
  - http://www.nsclc.org
- Nausea/Vomiting
  - http://www.aafp.org
  - http://www.acg.gi.org
  - http://www.acponline.org
  - http://www.gastro.org
- Neurological Disorders
  - http://www.aan.com
  - http://www.aanos.org
  - http://www.aesnet.org
  - http://www.neurosurgery.org
  - http://www.ninds.nih.gov
  - http://www.nmss.org
  - http://www.parkinson.org
- Neurofibromatosis/Von Recklinghausen Disease
  - http://www.aan.com
  - http://www.acponline.org
  - http://www.healthsystem.virginia.edu
  - http://www.meddhelp.org
  - http://www.ninds.nih.gov
- Neurological Surgery
  - http://www.aanos.org
  - http://www.aans.org
- Neuropathy
  - http://www.aafp.org

- http://www.aan.com
- http://www.acponline.org
- http://www.ninds.nih.gov
- Nervousness
  - http://www.aafp.org
  - http://www.nimh.nih.gov
  - http://www.nmha.org
- Nightmares/Children
  - http://www.aafp.org
  - http://www.aap.org
  - http://www.healthcare.ucla.edu
  - http://www.kidshealth.org
  - http://www.psych.org
- Nuclear Medicine
  - http://www.snm.org
- Nutrition/Dietary Guidelines
  - American College of Nutrition
    http://www.am-coll-nutr.org
  - Antioxidants and Alzheimer's Disease/Aging Prevention
    http://www.nia.nih.gov
  - Antioxidants and Cancer Prevention
    http://www.cancer.gov
  - Antioxidants and Heart Disease Prevention
    http://www.americanheart.org
  - Antioxidants and Macular Degeneration Prevention
    http://www.nei.nih.gov
  - Carbohydrate Intake/Recommendations
    http://www.hsph.harvard.edu/nutritionsource/carbohydrates.html
  - Center for Nutrition Policy Promotion
    http://www.usda.gov/cnpp
  - Dietary Guidelines
    http://www.americanheart.org
    http://www.cdc.gov/nccdphp/dnpa/site_index
    http://www.cyberdiet.org
    http://www.eatright.org
    http://www.usda.gov
  - Dietary Supplements
    http://www.ama-assn.org
    http://www.cfsan.fda.gov/~dms/ds-oview.html

http://www.cfsan.fda.gov/~dms/supplmnt.html
http://www.cfsan.fda.gov/~dms/fdsupp.html
http://www.ods.nih.gov
- Digestive Health and Nutrition Foundation
  http://www.fdhn.org
- Dr. Ornish Diet/Lifestyle Program
  http://www.webmd.com
- Fat Intake/Recommendations
  http://www.hsph.harvard.edu/nutritionsource/fats.html
- Fiber Intake/Recommendations
  http://www.hsph.harvard.edu/nutritionsource/fiber.html
- Food and Nutrition Board/Institute of Medicine
  http://www.iom.edu
- Food and Nutrition Information Center
  http://www.nal.usda.gov/fnic
- Food and Nutrition Intake/Recommendations
  http://www.ers.usda.gov/Briefing/DietandHealth
- Food Guide Pyramid
  http://www.usda.gov/cnpp
- Food Nutrient Data Laboratory
  http://www.nal.usda.gov/fnic/foodcomp
- Food Phytonutrient Laboratory
  http://www.barc.usda.gov/bhnrc/pl
- Food Pyramid: What Should You Eat
  http://www.hsph.harvard.edu/nutritionsource/pyramids.html
- Food Safety
  http://www.fda.gov
- Fruits and Vegetables: 5 to 9 a Day for Better Health
  http://www.cdc.gov/nccdphp/dnpa/5aday.whatis.htm
  http://www.cdc.gov/nccdphp/dnpa/5aday/faq
  http://www.cdc.gov/nccdphp/dnpa/tips/quick_tips.htm
  http://www.hsph.harvard.edu/nutritionsource/fruits.html
- General Information
  http://www.nutrition.org
- Interactive Health Eating Index
  http://www.usda.gov/cnpp
- International Food and Information Council
  http://www.ific.org

- Mediterranean Diet/Pyramid
    http://www.americanheart.org
    http://mayoclinic.com
- Mercury in Fish
    http://www.fda.gov
- Nutrition and Physical Activity
    http://www.cdc.gov/nccdphp/dnpa/site_index.htm
- Nutritional Sciences
    http://www.nutrition.org
- Phytonutrient/Phytochemical Content of Food
    http://www.nal.usda.gov/fnic/foodcom
- Protein Intake/Recommendations
    http://www.hsph.Harvard.edu/nutritionsource/protein.html
- Trans Fats Intake/Recommendations
    http://www.hsph.harvard.edu/reviews/transfats.html
- Tufts University Nutritional Navigator
    http://www.navigator.tufts.edu
- United Kingdom Food Standards
    http://www.foodstandards.gov.uk
- Vegetarian Diet
    http://www.vrg.org
- Vitamins and Minerals: How Much Do You Need
    http://www.fda.gov/fdac/special/foodlabel/dvs.html
    http://www.foodstandards.gov.uk
    http://www.iom.edu
    http://www.mayoclinic.com
    http://www.who.int

2.15 Obsessive-Compulsive Disorders to Overweight/Obesity

- Obsessive-Compulsive Disorders
    - http://www.aafp.org
    - http://www.adaa.org
    - http://www.mentalhelp.net
    - http://www.nami.org
    - http://www.nimh.nih.gov
    - http://www.nmha.org
    - http://www.psych.org

- Obstetrics/Gynecology
  - http://www.acog.org
- Occupational/Environmental Health/Safety
  - http://www.aafp.org
  - http://www.acoem.org
  - http://www.aiha.org
  - http://www.cdc.gov
  - http://www.osha.gov
- Oriental Medicine
  - http://www.acuall.org
  - http://www.hon.ch
  - http://www.intellihealth.com
  - http://www.medhelp.org
  - http://www.mayoclinic.com
  - http://www.nccam.nih.gov
  - http://www.webmd.com
- Orthopedic Surgery
  - http://www.aacs.org
  - http://www.aanos.org
  - http://www.clevelandclinic.org
- Orthostatic Hypotension
  - http://www.acc.org
  - http://www.acponline.org
  - http://www.americanheart.org
  - http://www.ninds.nih.gov
  - http://www.nhlbi.nih.org
- Osteoarthritis
  - http://www.aafp.org
  - http://www.arthritis.org
  - http://www.niams.nih.gov
- Osteomyelitis
  - http://www.aafp.org
  - http://www.acponline.org
  - http://www.niams.nih.gov
- Osteopathic Medicine
  - http://www.aoa-net.org/Consumers/consumers.htm
  - http://www.osteopathic.org

- Osteoporosis
  - http://www.aafp.org
  - http://www.4women
  - http://www.niams.nih.gov
  - http://www.nof.org
  - http://www.womenshealthmatters.ca
- Otitis Externa
  - http://www.aafp.org
  - http://www.entnet.org
- Otitis Media
  - http://www.aafp.org
  - http://www.aap.org
  - http://www.entnet.org
  - http://www.nidcd.nih.gov
- Otosclerosis
  - http://www.aafp.org
  - http://www.audiology.org
  - http://www.entnet.org
  - http://www.nidcd.nih.gov
  - http://www.mc.vanderbilt.edu
- Ovarian Cancer
  - http://www.cancer.gov
  - http://www.oncolink.upen.edu
  - http://www.ovarian.org
  - http://www.ovariancancer.org
- Overweight/Obesity/Health
  - Basics
    http://www.aafp.org
    http://www.asbs.org
    http://www.cdc.gov/nccdphp/dnpa
    http://www.nhlbi.nih.gov
    http://www.niddk.nih.gov
    http://www.obesity.org
    http://www.who.int
  - Body Mass Index
    http://www.cdc.gov/nccdphp/dnpa/bmi-means.htm
    http://www.cdc.gov/nccdphp/dnpa/bmi/bmi-adult.htm
    http://www.nhlbi.nih.gov/guidelines/obesity/bmi_tbl.htm

- Clinical Guidelines on the Identification, Evaluation and Treatment of Overweight and Obesity in Adults
  http://www.nhlbi.nih.gov/guidelines/obesity/ob_home.htm
  http://www.nhlbi.nih.gov/guidelines/obesity/sum_evid.htm
- Do you Know the Health Risks of Being Overweight
  http://www.niddk.nih.gov/health/nutrit/pubs/health.htm
- Overweight and Obesity Overview
  http://www.cdc.gov/nccdphjp/dnpa/obestiy/index.htm
- **Overweight/Obesity/Weight Loss Program**
  - Aim for a Healthy Weight: Key Recommendations
    http://www.nhlbi.nih.gov/health/public/heart/obesity/lose-wt/recommen.htm
  - Assessing Your Risk
    http://www.nhlbi.nih.gov/health/public/heart/obesity/lose-wt/risk.htm
  - Drug Therapy for Obesity
    http://www.aafp.org/afp/20000615/3615/html
  - Guide to Behavior Change
    http://www.nhlbi.nih.gov/health/public/heart/obesity/lose_wt/behavior.htm
  - Medical Management of Obesity
    http://www.aafp.org/afp/20000715/419.html
  - Prescription Medications for the Treatment of Obesity
    http://www.niddk.nih.gov/health/nutrit/pubs/presmeds.htm
  - Selecting a Weight Loss Program
    http://www.nhlbi.nih.gov/health/public/heart/obesity/lose_wt/wtl_prog.htm
  - Weight Loss Tips
    http://www.nhlbi.nih.gov/health/public/heart/obesity/lose_wt/ob_tips.htm
- **Overweight/Obesity/Surgical Treatment**
  - Gastric Bypass Surgery for Severe Obesity
    http://www.niddk.nih.gov/health/nutrit/pubs/gastsurg.htm
  - Rational for the Treatment of Morbid (Severe) Obesity
    http://www.asbs.org/html/rationale/rationale.html
    http://www.yoursurgery.com

2.16 Pain Management to Pyelonephritis

- Pain/Management
  - http://www.aafp/org
  - http://www.aanhfp.org
  - http://www.ampainsoc.org
  - http://www.druginfonet.com

- http://www.fda.gov
- http://www.painfoundation.org
- http://www.painmed.org
- Paget's Disease/Bone
  - http://www.aafp.org
  - http://www.healthcare.ucla.edu
  - http://www.niams.nih.gov
  - http://www.paget.org
- Palpitations
  - http://www.aafp.org
  - http://www.acc.org
  - http://www.americanheart.org
- Pancreatitis
  - http://www.acg.gi.org
  - http://www.acponline.org
  - http://www.gastro.org
  - http://www.medhelp.org
- Panic Disorder
  - http://www.aafp.org
  - http://www.mentalhelp.net
  - http://www.nimh.nih.gov
  - http://www.nmha.org
  - http://www.psych.org
- PAP/Papanicolaou Smear/Test
  - http://www.aafp.org
  - http://www.acog.org
  - http://www.cytopathology.org
- Paralysis
  - http://www.aafp.org
  - http://www.ninds.nih.gov
  - http://www.stroke.org
- Parasitic Infections
  - http://www.aafp.org
  - http://www.acponline.org
  - http://www.aphl.org
  - http://www.cdc.gov
  - http://www.niaid.nih.gov
- Parathyroid Disease
  - http://www.aace.com/college

- http://www.acponline.org
- http://www.healthcare.ucla.edu
- http://www.medhelp.org
- Parenting Tips
  - http://www.aafp.org
  - http;//www.aap.org
  - http;//www.ama-assn.org
  - http://www.kidshealth.org
- Parkinson's Disease
  - http://www.aafp.org
  - http://www.aan.com
  - http://www.apdaparkinson.com
  - http://www.healthcare.ucla.edu
  - http://www.ninds.nih.gov
  - http://www.parkinson.org
  - http://www.pdf.org
- Paronychia/Finger/Toe Infection
  - http://www.aad.org
  - http://www.aafp.org
  - http://www.apma.org
  - http://www.heathcare.ucla.edu
  - http://www.healthsysstem.virginia.edu
- Patient Advocacy
  - http://www.ama-assn.org
  - http://www.canceradvocacy.org
  - http://www.patientadvocate.org
- Pediatric Disorders
  - http://www.aafp.org
  - http://www.aap.org
  - http://www.kidshealth.org
  - http://www.nichd.nih.gov
- Pediculosis
  - http://www.aad.org
  - http://www.aafp.org
  - http://www.aap.org
  - http://www.cdc.gov
  - http://www.kidshealth.org
- Pelvic Inflammatory Disease
  - http://www.aafp.org
  - http://www.acog.org

- Peptic Ulcer
  - http://www.aafp.org
  - http://www.acg.gi.org
  - http://www.gastro.org
  - http://www.niddk.nih.gov
- Pericarditis
  - http://www.acc.org
  - http://www.acponline.org
  - http://www.americanheart.org
  - http://www.nhlbi.nih.gov
- Peripheral Vascular Disease
  - http://www.aafp.org
  - http://www.acponline.org
  - http://www.healthcare.ucla.edu
  - http://www.nhlbi.nih.gov
  - http://www.scvir.org
- Personality Disorder
  - http://www.apa.org
  - http://www.mentalhelp.net
  - http://www.nmha.org
  - http://www.psych.org
- Pes Planus/Flat Feet
  - http://www.aafp.org
  - http://www.aofas.org
  - http://www.apma.org
- Petechiae
  - http://www.aafp.org
  - http://www.acponline.org
  - http://www.hematology.org
  - http://www.nhlbi.nih.gov
- Pharyngitis
  - http://www.aafp.org
  - http://www.aap.org
  - http://www.entnet.org
- Pheochromocytoma
  - http://www.aace.com/college
  - http://www.acponline.org
  - http://www.cancer.gov

- Phimosis/Penis
  - http://www.aafp.org
  - http://www.aap.org
  - http://www.acog.org
- Phobias
  - http://www.apa.org
  - http://www.mentalhelp.net
  - http://www.nimh.nih.gov
  - http://www.nmha.org
  - http://www.psych.org
- Photorefractive Keratectomy
  - http://www.aao.org
  - http://www.ascrs.org
  - http://www.nei.nih.gov
- Physical Abuse
  - http://www.aafp.org
  - http://www.cdc.gov
  - http://www.elderabusecenter.org
  - http://www.kidshealth.org
- Physical Activity/Exercise/Fitness/Health
  - American College of Sports Medicine
    http://www.acsm.org
  - American Hiking Association
    http://www.americanhiking.org
  - American Medical Association
    http://www.ama-assn.org
  - Efit
    http://www.efit.com
  - Global Health and Fitness
    http://www.global-fitness.com
  - Great Outdoors Recreation Page
    http://www.gorp.com
  - Guide to Physical Activity
    http://www.nhlbi.nih.gov/health/public/heart/obesity/lose_wt/phy_act.htm
  - Just Move
    http://www.justmove.org
  - Kids Health
    http://www.kidshealth.org

- National Center for Chronic Disease Prevention and Health Promotion
  http://www.cdc.gov/nccdphp/dnpa
- National Wellness Institute
  http://www.nationalwellness.org
- Net Wellness
  http://www.netwellness.org
- Outdoors.org
  http://www.outdoors.org
- Physical Activity Recommendations
  http://www.cdc.gov/nccdphp/dnpa/physical/recommendations.htm
- President's Council on Physical fitness and Sports
  http://www.fitness.gov
- Promoting Active Lifestyle Among Older Adults
  http://www.cdc.gov/nccdphp/dnpa/physical/lifestyles.htm
- Recreation.gov
  http://www.recreation.gov
- Shape Up America
  http://www.shapeup.org
- World Health Organization
  http://www.who.int

■ Physical Therapy/Rehabilitation
  - http://www.aapmr.org
  - http://www.apta.org
  - http://www.healthsystem.virginia.edu

■ Physicans/Professional Organizations
  - http://www.ama-assn.org
  - http://www.healthfinder.gov
  - http://www.wedmd.com

■ Pilonidal Cyst
  - http://www.aafp.org
  - http://www.facrs.org

■ Pinworm Infection
  - http://www.aafp.org
  - http://www.aap.org
  - http://www.cdc.gov
  - http://www.kidshealth.org

■ Pityriasis Rosea
  - http://www.aad.org
  - http://www.aafp.org
  - http://www.niams.nih.gov

- Plague
  - http://www.acponline.org
  - http://www.cdc.gov
  - http://www.medhelp.org
  - http://www.niaid.nih.gov
  - http://www.who.int
- Planned Parenthood
  - http://www.ppfa.org
- Plantar Fascitis/Foot
  - http://www.aaos.org
  - http://www.aofas.org
  - http://www.apma.org
- Plantar Wart/Foot
  - http://www.aafp.org
  - http://www.apma.org
  - http://www.healthsystem.virginia.edu
  - http://www.noah-health.org
- Plastic/Reconstructive Surgery
  - http://www.facial-plastic-surgery.org
  - http://www.plasticsurgery.rog
- Pleurisy
  - http://www.aafp.org
  - http://www.acponline.org
  - http://www.chestnet.org
  - http://www.nhlbi.nih.gov
- Pneumonia
  - http://www.aafp.org
  - http://www.acponline.org
  - http://www.cdc.gov
  - http://www.chestnet.org
  - http://www.nhlbi.nih.gov
- Pneumonia Prevention/Elderly
  - http://www.aafp.org
  - http://www.americangeriatrics.org
  - http://www.cdc.gov
  - http://www.chestnet.org
  - http://www.nia.nih.gov
- Pneumothorax
  - http://www.aafp.org

- http://www.acep.com
- http://www.acponline.org
- Poison Control Centers
  - http://www.aapcc.org
  - http://www.aphl.org
- Poisoning/Chemical
  - http://www.aafp.org
  - http://www.aap.org
  - http://www.aapcc.org
  - http://www.acep.com
  - http://www.aphl.org
  - http://www.cdc.gov/niosh
- Poliomyelitis/Vaccination
  - http://www.aafp.org
  - http://www.aap.org
  - http://www.cdc.gov
  - http://www.niaid.nih.gov
  - http://www.who.int
- Polycythemia
  - http://www.acponline.org
  - http://www.clevelandclinic.org
  - http://www.healthsystem.virginia.edu
  - http://www.hematology.org
  - http://www.nhlbi.nih.gov
- Polymyalgia Rheumatica
  - http://www.arthritis.org
  - http://www.clevelandclinic.org
  - http://www.healthsystem.virginia.edu
  - http://www.rheumatology.org
- Post Nasal Drip
  - http://www.aafp.org
  - http://www.entnet.org
- Post Traumatic Stress Disorder
  - http://www.aafp.org
  - http://www.apa.org
  - http://www.mentalhelp.net
  - http://www.ncptsd.org
  - http://www.nimh.nih.gov
  - http://www.nmha.org

- http://www.psych.org
- http://www.ptsdalliance.org
- PPD/Tuberculosis Test
  - http://www.aafp.org
  - http://www.acponline.org
  - http://www.chestnet.org
- Practice/Treatment Guidelines
  - http://www.ama-assn.org
  - http://www.guideline.gov
- Pregnancy
  - http://www.aafp.org
  - http://www.acog.org
  - http://www.ama-assn.org
- Premenstral Tension Syndrome
  - http://www.acog.org
  - http://www.4women.gov
  - http://www.womenshealthmatters.ca
- Presbycusis/Aging Hearing Loss
  - http://www.americangeriatrics.org
  - http://www.aoa.dhhs.gov
  - http://www.nia.nih.gov
- Prescription/OTC Drug Information
  - http://www.druginfonet.com
  - http://www.fda.gov
  - http://www.fda.gov/oc/buyonline
  - http://www.fda.gov/cder
  - http://www.rxlist.com
- Pressure Sore/Decubitus Ulcer
  - http://www.aafp.org
  - http://www.ama-assn.org
  - http://www.americangeriatrics.org
  - http://www.medhelp.org
- Preventive Medicine
  - http://www.acpm.org
  - http://www.aphl.org
  - http://www.americanshealth.org
  - http://www.aspo.org
  - http://www.cdc.gov
  - http://www.iom.edu

- Proctitis
  - http://www.aafp.org
  - http://www.acg.gi.org
  - http://www.niddk.nih.gov
- Prostate Disease
  - http://www.aafp.org
  - http://www.afud.org
  - http://www.auanet.org
  - http://www.niddk.nih.gov
  - http://www.prostateinfo.com
- Pruritis/Itching Skin/Anus
  - http://www.aad.org
  - http://www.aafp.org
  - http://www.fascrs.org
- Psoriasis
  - http://www.aad.org
  - http://www.aafp.org
  - http://www.clevelandclinic.org
  - http://www.psoriasis.org
- Psychiatry
  - http://www.aacap.org
  - http://www.aacp.com
  - http://www.mentalhelp.net
  - http://www.nimh.nih.gov
  - http://www.psych.org
- Psychology/Counseling
  - http://www.aacp.org
  - http://www.apa.org
  - http://www.cyberpsych.org
  - http://www.mentalhelp.net
- Psychosomatic Disorders
  - http://www.apa.org
  - http://www.apm.org
  - http://www.mbmi.org
  - http://www.psych.org
  - http://www.psychosomatic.org
- Ptosis/Drooping Eyelid
  - http://www.aafp.org
  - http://www.aao.org

- Public Health
  - http://www.aphl.org
  - http://www.cdc.gov
  - http://www.os.dhhs.gov
  - http://www.surgeongeneral.gov
- Pulmonary Edema
  - http://www.aafp.org
  - http://www.acc.org
  - http://www.acponline.org
  - http://www.nhlbi.nih.gov
- Pulmonary Hypertension
  - http://www.acc.org
  - http://www.acponline.org
  - http://www.nhlbi.nih.gov
- Pulmonary Value Stenosis
  - http://www.acc.org
  - http://www.acponline.org
  - http://www.americanheart.org
  - http://www.nhlbi.nih.gov
- Pylonephritis
  - http://www.aafp.org
  - http://www.acponline.org
  - http://www.kidney.org
  - http://www.niddk.nih.gov

2.17 Quality HealthCare/Research

- Quality Healthcare/Research
  - http://www.ahrq.gov
  - http://www.ama-assn.org
  - http://www.who.int

2.18 Rabies/Vaccination to Rubella/German Measles

- Rabies/Vaccination
  - http://www.afp.org
  - http://www.acponline

- http://www.cdc.gov
- http://www.who.int
- **Radiation Therapy**
  - http://www.acr.org
  - http://www.astro.org
  - http://www.clevelandclinic.org
  - http://www.noah-health.org
- **Radiology**
  - http://www.acr.org
  - http://www.astro.org
  - http://www.sirweb.org
- **Rape**
  - http://www.aafp.org
  - http://www.cdc.gov
  - http://www.4women.gov
  - http://www.womens-health.org
  - http://www.womenshealthmatters.ca
- **Rare Diseases**
  - http://www.hon.ch
  - http://www.rarediseases.info.nih.gov/ord
- **Rash/Skin**
  - http://www.aad.org
  - http://www.aafp.org
  - http://www.aap.org
  - http://www.acfp.org
- **Raynaud's Syndrome**
  - http://www.aafp.org
  - http://www.acc.org
  - http://www.acponline.org
  - http://www.clevelandclinic.org
  - http://www.nhlbi.nih.gov
  - http://www.niams.nih.gov
- **Rectal Prolapse/Bleeding**
  - http://www.acg.gi.org
  - http://www.facrs.org
  - http://www.gastro.org
- **Reflex Sympathetic Dystrophy**
  - http://www.aan.com
  - http://www.healthsystem.virginia.edu

- http://www.medhelp.org
- http://www.ninds.nih.gov
- **Refractive Errors Eye/Surgery**
  - http://www.aao.org
  - http://www.ascrs.org
  - http://www.isrs.org
  - http://www.lasikinstitute.org
  - http://www.nei.nih.gov
  - http://www.preventblindness.org
- **Reiter's Syndrome**
  - http://www.aafp.org
  - http://www.acponline.org
  - http://www.medhelp.org
  - http://www.niams.nih.gov
  - http://www.webmd.com
- **Reproductive Medicine**
  - http://www.acog.org
  - http://www.arhp.org
  - http://www.asrm.org
  - http://www.ivf.org
  - http://www.maleinfertility.org
- **Respiratory Care**
  - http://www.aafp.org
  - http://www.aarc.org
  - http://www.chestnet.org
  - http://www.lungusa.org
  - http://www.nhlbi.nih.gov
- **Respiratory Distress Syndrome**
  - http://www.chestnet.org
  - http://www.cdc.gov
  - http://www.lungusa.org
  - http://www.nhlbi.nih.gov
- **Respiratory Infections/Upper/Lower**
  - http://www.aafp.org
  - http://www.chestnut.org
  - http://www.nhlbi.nih.gov
- **Restless Legs Syndrome**
  - http://www.aafp.org
  - http://www.aan.com

- http://www.healthsystem.virginia.edu
- http://www.ninds.nih.gov
- **Retinal Detachment**
  - http://www.aao.org
  - http://www.diabetes.org
  - http://www.eyenet.org
  - http://www.nei.nih.gov
  - http://www.preventblindness.org
- **Retinopathy**
  - http://www.aao.org
  - http://www.diabetes.org
  - http://www.eyenet.org
  - http://www.nei.nih.gov
  - http://www.preventblindness.org
- **Rheumatic Heart Disease**
  - http://www.aafp.org
  - http://www.acc.org
  - http://www.americanheart.org
  - http://www.nhlbi.nih.gov
- **Rheumatoid Arthritis/Disorders**
  - http://www.arthritis.org
  - http://www.clevelandclinic.org
  - http://www.medhelp.org
  - http://www.niams.nih.gov
  - http://www.rheumatology.org
- **Rhinitis**
  - http://www.aaaai.org
  - http://www.aafp.org
  - http://www.entnet.org
  - http;//www.niaid.nih.gov
- **Rickets**
  - http://www.aafp.org
  - http://www.aap.org
  - http://www.kidshealth.org
- **Ringworm/Tinea Corporis**
  - http://www.aafp.org
  - http://www.aap.org
  - http://www.kidshelath.org

- Rocky Mountain Spotted Fever
  - http://www.aafp.org
  - http://www.acponline.org
  - http://www.cdc.gov
- Rosacea
  - http://www.aad.org
  - http://www.aafp.org
  - http://www.niams.nih.gov
- Rotator Cuff Disorder/Tear
  - http://www.aafp.org
  - http://www.aaos.org
  - http://www.niams.nih.gov
- Rubella/German Measles
  - http://www.aafp.org
  - http://www.aap.org
  - http://www.cdc.gov
  - http://www.kidshealth.org
  - http://www.nfid.org

2.19 Salmonella Gastroenteritis to Systemic Lupus

- Salmonella Gastroenteritis
  - http://www.aafp.org
  - http://www.acg.gi.org
  - http://www.acponline.org
  - http://www.aphl.org
  - http://www.cdc.gov
- Sarcoidosis
  - http://www.aafp.org
  - http://www.acponline.org
  - http://www.clevelandclinic.org
  - http://www.nhlbi.nih.gov
- SARS/Sudden Acute Respiratory Syndrome
  - http://www.aphl.org
  - http://www.cdc.gov
  - http://www.chestnet.org
  - http://www.lungusa.org
  - http://www.niaid.nih.gov
  - http://www.who.int

- Scabies
  - http://www.aad.org
  - http://www.aafp.org
  - http://www.cdc.gov
  - http://www.kidshealth.org
- Schizophrenia
  - http://www.mentalhelp.net
  - http://www.nami.org
  - http://www.nimh.nih.gov
  - http://www.nmha.org
  - http://www.psych.org
- Scleroderma
  - http://www.aad.org
  - http://www.aafp.org
  - http://www.acponline.org
  - http://www.healthcare.ucla.edu
  - http://www.healthsystem.virginia.edu
  - http://www.scleroderma.org
- Scoliosis
  - http://www.aafp.org
  - http://www.aaos.org
  - http://www.aap.org
  - http://www.niams.nih.gov
- Seborrheic Dermatitis
  - http://www.aad.org
  - http://www.aafp.org
- Seborrheic Keratosis
  - http://www.aad.org
  - http://www.aafp.org
- Seeing Impaired
  - http://www.aao.org
  - http://www.afb.org
  - http://www.lighthouse.org
  - http://www.preventblindness.org
- Senile Dementia
  - http://www.aafp.org
  - http://www.americangeriatrics.org
  - http://www.geron.org
  - http://www.nia.nih.gov

- Senior Health
    - http://www.ama-assn.org
    - http://www.americangeriatrics.org
    - http://www.geron.org
    - http://www.intellihealth.com
    - http://www.mayoclinic.com
    - http://www.noah-health.org
    - http://www.nslc.org
    - http://www.webmd.com
- Sexual Dysfunction
    - http://www.aafp.org
    - http://www.afud.org
    - http://www.asrm.org
    - http://www.noah-health.org
- Sexually Transmitted Diseases
    - http://www.aafp.org
    - http://www.aphl.org
    - http://www.ashastd.org
    - http://www.cdc.gov
    - http://www.healthydevil.studentaffairs.duke.edu
    - http://www.medweb.emory.edu/medweb/
    - http://www.niaid.nih.gov
- Shigellosis
    - http://www.aafp.org
    - http://www.aphl.org
    - http://www.cdc.gov
    - http://www.nfid.org
- Shortness of Breath
    - http://www.aafp.org
    - http://www.acc.org
    - http://www.acponline.org
    - http://www.chestnet.org
- Shoulder Dislocation/Separation
    - http://www.aafp.org
    - http://www.aaos.org
    - http://www.acep.com
    - http://www.niams.nih.gov
- Shoulder/Frozen
    - http://www.aafp.org

- http://www.aanos.org
- http://www.aaos.org
- http://www.niams.nih.gov
- Sickle Cell Disease
  - http://www.aspho.org
  - http://www.healthcare.ulca.edu
  - http://www.hematology.org
  - http://www.nhlbi.nihgov
- Sigmoidoscopy
  - http://www.aafp.org
  - http://www.acg.gi.org
  - http://www.gastro.org
  - http://www.sages.org
- Sinusitis
  - http://www.aafp.org
  - http://www.entnet.org
- Sjogren's Disease
  - http://www.acponline.org
  - http://www.clevelandclinic.org
  - http://www.healthcare.ucla.edu
  - http://www.healthsystem.virginia.edu
  - http://www.sjogrens.com
- Skin Cancer Treatments
  - http://www.aad.org
  - http://www.asds-net.org
  - http://www.cancer.gov
- Skin Care/Elderly
  - http://www.aad.org
  - http://www.aafp.org
  - http://www.americangeriatrics.org
  - http://www.nia.nih.gov
- Skin Disorders/Nevi/Moles/Tags
  - http://www.aad.org
  - http://www.aafp.org
  - http://www.asds-net.org
  - http://www.cancernet.nci.nih.gov
  - http://www.mohscollege.org
  - http://www.niams.nih.gov
  - http://www.psoriasis.org

- **Skin Resurfacing/Laser**
  - http://www.aad.org
  - http://www.aafp.org
  - http://www.asds-net.org
- **Sleep Apnea**
  - http://www.acponline.org
  - http://www.healthsystem.virginia.edu
  - http://www.medhelp.org
  - http://www.sleepfoundation.org
- **Sleep Disorders**
  - http://www.aafp.org
  - http://www.aasmnet.org
  - http://www.intellihealth.com
  - http://www.mayoclinic.com
  - http://www.medhelp.org
  - http://www.nhlbi.nih.gov/about/ncsdr/index.htm
  - http://www.sleepfoundation.org
  - http://www.webmd.com
- **Smallpox/Variola**
  - http://www.bt.cdc.gov
  - http://www.medhelp.org
  - http://www.niaid.nih.gov
  - http://www.webmd.com
  - http://www.who.int
- **Smoking Related Disorders**
  - http://www.ama-assn.org
  - http://www.cdc.gov
  - http://www.chestnet.org
  - http://www.lungusa.org
  - http://www.who.int
- **Snoring**
  - http://www.aafp.org
  - http://www.entnet.org
  - http://www.medhelp.org
  - http://www.webmd.com
- **Social Phobia**
  - http://www.adaa.org
  - http://www.apa.org
  - http://www.nimh.nih.gov

- http://www.nmha.org
- http://www.psych.org
- Soft Tissue Augmentation
  - http://www.aad.org
  - http://www.asds-net.org
  - http://www.clevelandclinic.org
  - http://www.healthcare.ucla.edu
- Somnambulism
  - http://www.aafp.org
  - http://www.aap.org
  - http://www.healthcare.ucla.edu
  - http://www.sleepfoundation.org
- Spasticity/Extremity
  - http://www.aan.com
  - http://www.ninds.nih.gov
- Spider Veins
  - http://www.aad.org
  - http://www.aafp.org
- Spina Bifida
  - http://www.aap.org
  - http://www.healthcare.ucla.edu
  - http://www.kidshealth.org
  - http://www.sbaa.org
- Spinal Health/Stenosis
  - http://www.aafp.org
  - http://www.aan.com
  - http://www.aanos.org
  - http://www.spine-health.com
- Spirituality and Health
  - http://www.aafp.org
  - http://www.ama-assn.org
  - http://www.dukespiritualityandhealth.org/
  - http://www.gwish.org
  - http://www.kidshealth.org
- Spondylosis
  - http://www.aaos.org
  - http://www.arthritis.org
  - http://www.niams.nih.gov

- Sports Injury
  - http://www.aaos.org
  - http://www.acsm.org
- Sports Medicine
  - http://www.aafp.org
  - http://www.ama-assn.org
  - http://www.acsm.org
- Sprain/Strain
  - http://www.aafp.org
  - http://www.aaos.org
- Stem Cells/Transplantation
  - http://www.cancer.gov
  - http://www.clinicaltrials.gov
  - http://www.health.nih.gov
  - http://www.niaid.nih.gov
  - http://www.nlm.nih.gov
  - http://www.stemcellresearchfoundation.org
  - http://www.who.int
- Strabismus/Lazy Eye Syndrome/Amblyopia
  - http://www.aao.org
  - http://www.preventblindess.org
  - http://www.nei.nih.gov
- Strep Throat
  - http://www.aafp.org
  - http://www.aap.org
  - http://www.entnet.org
  - http://www.niaid.nih.gov
- Stress Incontinence
  - http://www.acog.org
  - http://www.auanet.org
  - http://www.niddk.nih.gov
- Stress/Psychological
  - http://www.aafp.org
  - http://www.apa.org
  - http://www.mbmi.org
  - http://www.mentalhelp.net
  - http://www.nmha.org
  - http://www.psychosomatic.org
  - http://www.stress.org
  - http://www.umassmed.edu/cfm

- Stroke
  - http://www.aafp.org
  - http://www.acc.org
  - http://www.acponline.org
  - http://www.americanheart.org
  - http://www.ninds.nih.gov
  - http://www.stroke.org
- Student Health
  - http://www.aafp.org
  - http://www.healthcare.ucla.edu
  - http://www.healthsystem.virginia.edu
  - http://www.healthydevil.studentaffairs.duke.edu
  - http://www.medweb.emory.edu/medweb/
- Stuttering
  - http://www.apa.org
  - http://www.mentalhelp.net
  - http://www.nidcd.nih.gov
  - http://www.psych.org
- Stye/Hordoleum
  - http://www.aafp.org
  - http://www.aao.org
  - http://www.eyenet.org
- Substance Abuse
  - http://www.aafp.orgh
  - http://www.aap.org
  - http://www.nida.nih.gov
  - http://www.nmha.org
  - http://www.psych.org
- Sudden Infant Death Syndrome
  - http://www.aafp.org
  - http://www.aap.org
  - http://www.mc.vanderbilt.edu
- Suicide Prevention
  - http://www.acpm.org
  - http://www.cdc.gov
  - http://www.mentalhelp.net
  - http://www.psych.org
  - http://www.suicidology.org

- Sunburn
  - http://www.aad.org
  - http://www.aafp.org
  - http://www.intellihealth.com
  - http://www.webmd.com
- Surgery
  - http://www.aanos.org
  - http://www.aans.org
  - http://www.aao.org
  - http://www.acsm.org
  - http://www.asds_net.org
  - http://www.facial_plastic_surgery.org
  - http://www.facs.org
  - http://www.hand_surgery.org
  - http://www.mohscollege.org
  - http://www.neurosurgery.org
  - http://www.sages.org
  - http://www.skincancerinfo.com
  - http://www.yoursurgery
- Sweating Excessively/Hyperhidrosis
  - http://www.aad.org
  - http://www.aafp.org
  - http://www.acponline.org
  - http://www.niams.nih.gov
  - http://www.sweathelp.org
- Syncope
  - http://www.aafp.org
  - http://www.acponline.org
  - http://www.americanheart.org
  - http://www.ninds.nih.gov
- Syphilis
  - http://www.cdc.gov
  - http://www.healthsystem.virginia.edu
  - http://www.niaid.nih.gov
  - http://www.who.int
- Systemic Lupus Erythematous
  - http://www.aarda.org
  - http://www.healthcare.ucla.edu
  - http://www.healthsystem.virginia.edu
  - http://www.lupus.org

2.20 Tachycardia to Tularemia

- Tachycardia/Rapid Heart Beat
  - http://www.aafp.org
  - http://www.acc.org
  - http://www.acponline.org
  - http://www.americanheart.org
- Teeth Grinding/Bruxism/TMJ Syndrome
  - http://www.aafp.org
  - http://www.ada.org
  - http://www.entent.org
  - http://www.mayoclinic.com
- Tennis Elbow
  - http://www.aafp.org
  - http://www.aaos.org
- Tenosynovitis/DeQuervan's Syndrome
  - http://www.aafp.org
  - http://www.aaos.org
- Thyroid Disease
  - http://www.aafp.org
  - http://www.acponline.org
  - http://www.the-thyroid-society.org
  - http://www.thyroid.org
  - http://www.tsh.org
- Thyroid Function Tests
  - http://www.labtestsonline.org
- Tick Borne Disease
  - http://www.aafp.org
  - http://www.acponline.org
  - http://www.cdc.org
  - http://www.kidshealth.org
- Tinea Versicolor/Eichstedt's Disease/Skin
  - http://www.aad.org
  - http://www.aafp.org
  - http://www.aap.org
- Tinnitus
  - http://www.aafp.org
  - http://www.ata.org
  - http://www.entnet.org

- **Tonsil/Adenoid Disease**
  - http://www.aafp.org
  - http://www.aap.org
  - http://www.entnet.org
- **Torticollis**
  - http://www.aafp.org
  - http://www.aap.org
  - http://www.torticollis.org
- **Toxic Shock Syndrome**
  - http://www.aafp.org
  - http://www.acponline.org
  - http://www.cdc.gov
- **Transient Ischemic Attack/TIA**
  - http://www.aafp.org
  - http://www.acponline.org
  - http://www.americanheart.org
  - http://www.ninds.nih.gov
  - http://www.stroke.org
- **Transplantation/Organ**
  - http://www.ishlt.org
  - http://www.niaid.nih.gov
- **Travel Health**
  - http://www.aafp.org
  - http://www.cdc.gov/travel
  - http://www.tripprep.com
- **Tremor**
  - http://www.aafp.org
  - http://www.ninds.nih.gov
  - http://www.webmd.com
- **Trichinosis**
  - http://www.aafp.org
  - http://www.acponline.org
  - http://www.cdc.gov
  - http://www.healthlink.mcw.edu
- **Trichotillomania/Compulsive Hair Pulling**
  - http://www.aad.org
  - http://www.aafp.org
  - http://www.mayoclinic.com

- http://www.psych.org
- http://www.trich.org
- Trigeminal Neuralgia
  - http://www.aafp.org
  - http://www.aan.com
  - http://www.ninds.nih.gov
- Trigger Finger
  - http://www.aafp.org
  - http://www.aaos.org
- Tropical Disease/Hygiene
  - http://www.aafp.org
  - http://www.ama-assn.org
  - http://www.astmh.org
  - http://www.cdc.gov
  - http://www.healthcare.ucla.edu
- Tuberculosis
  - http://www.aafp.org
  - http://www.acponline.org
  - http://www.aphl.org
  - http://www.cdc.gov
  - http://www.healthcare.ucla.edu
  - http://www.niaid.nih.gov
  - http://www.who.int
- Tularemia
  - http://www.aafp.org
  - http://www.acponline.org
  - http://www.cdc.gov
  - http://www.healthsystem.virginia.edu

2.21 Urethritis to Uterine Fibroids/Leiomyomas

- Urethritis
  - http://www.aafp.org
  - http://www.auanet.org
  - http://www.nfid.org
  - http://www.niaid.nih.gov
- Urinary Tract Disease
  - http://www.aafp.org
  - http://www.acponline.org

- http://www.afud.org
- http://www.auanet.org
- http://www.kidney.org
- http://www.nafc.org
- http://www.niddk.nih.gov
- http://www.prostrateinfo.com
- Urticaria
  - http://www.aad.org
  - http://www.aafp.org
- Uterine Fibroids/Leiomyomas
  - http://www.acog.org
  - http://www.facs.org
  - http://www.healthcare.ucla.edu
  - http://www.4women.org

2.22 Vaccines/Immunization to Vitiligo/Skin Depigmentation

- Vaccines/Immunization Schedules
  - http://www.aafp.org
  - http://www.acpm.org
  - http://www.ama-assn.org
  - http://www.cdc.gov
  - http://www.tripprep.com
- Vaginal Disorders/Bleeding/Discharge
  - http://www.aafp.org
  - http://www.acog.org
  - http://www.4women.gov
  - http://www.niaid.nih.gov
- Variocele/Scrotal
  - http://www.aafp.org
  - http://www.aap.org
  - http://www.facs.org
- Varicose Veins/Leg Ulcer
  - http://www.aafp.org
  - http://www.acponline.org
  - http://www.asds-net.org
  - http://www.intellihealth.com
  - http://www.mayoclinic.com

- Vertigo/Dizziness
  - http://www.aafp.org
  - http://www.aan.org
  - http://www.webmd.com
- Veterans Health
  - http://www.noah-health.org
  - http://www.va.org
  - http://www1.va.gov/health_benefits
- Violence Prevention
  - http://www.aafp.org
  - http://www.acog.org
  - http://www.cdc.gov
- Vision Disorders
  - http://www.aafp.org
  - http://www.aao.org
  - http://www.ascrs.org
  - http://www.lasikinstitute.org
  - http://www.nei.nih.gov
  - http://www.preventblindness.org
- Vitamins/Minerals
  - http://www.acpm.org
  - http://www.ama-assn.org
  - http://www.foodstandards.gov.uk
  - http://www.mayoclinic.com
  - http://www.wellweb.com
- Vitiligo/Skin Depigmentation
  - http://www.aad.org
  - http://www.aafp.org
  - http://www.healthsystem.virginia.edu
  - http://www.niams.nih.gov

2.23 Warts to Wounds

- Warts/Skin/Anal
  - http://www.aafp.org
  - http://www.cdc.gov
  - http://www.fascrs.org
- Waterborne Diseases
  - http://www.acpm.org

- http://www.ama-assn.org
- http://www.aphl.org
- http://www.cdc.gov
- http://www.who.int
- **Weakness/Fatigue**
  - http://www.aafp.org
  - http://www.acponline.org
- **Wellness**
  - http://www.ama-assn.org
  - http://www.nationalwellness.org
  - http://www.netwellness.org
  - http://www.wellness-community.org
- **West Nile Virus Disease**
  - http://www.aafp.org
  - http://www.acponline.org
  - http://www.aphl.org
  - http://www.cdc.gov
  - http://www.niaid.nih.gov
- **Women's Health**
  - http://www.aafp.org
  - http://www.anwa-doc.org
  - http://www.cdc.gov
  - http://www.fda.gov/womens/default.htm
  - http://www.4women.org
  - http://www.healthywomen.org
  - http://www.intellihealth.com
  - http://www.mayoclinic.com
  - http://www.menopause.org
  - http://www.noah-health.org
  - http://www.womens-health.org
  - http://www.womenshealthmatters.ca
- **Wound/Gunshot**
  - http://www.acep.com
  - http://www.cdc.gov
- **Wounds**
  - http://www.aafp.org
  - http://www.cdc.gov
  - http://www.facs.org

Chapter 3

Author's List/Key Web Health Resources/Websites

Academy of Psychosomatic Medicine
http://www.apm.org

Acoustic Neuroma Association
http://www.anausa.org

Administration on Aging
http://www.aoa.dhhs.gov

Agency for Healthcare Research and Quality
http://www.ahrq.gov

Alcoholics Anonymous
http://www.alcoholics-anonymous.org

All the Web
http://www.alltheweb.com

Alternative Medicine Homepage
http://www.pitt.edu/~cbw.altm.html

Alzheimer's Association
http://www.alz.org

Alzheimer's Disease Education and Referral Center
http://www.alzheimers.org

Alzheimer's Research Foundation
http://www.alzheimers-research.org

American Academy of Allergy, Asthma and Immunology
http://www.aaaai.org

American Academy of Audiology
http://www.audiology.org

American Academy for Cerebral Palsy and Developmental Medicine
http://www.aacpdm.org

American Academy of Child and Adolescent Psychiatry
http://www.aacap.org

American Academy of Clinical Psychiatrists
http://www.aacp.com

American Academy of Dermatology
http://www.aad.org

American Academy of Disability Evaluating Physicians
http://www.aadep.org

American Academy of Facial Plastic and Reconstructive Surgery
http://www.facial-plastic-surgery.org

American Academy of Family Physicians
http://www.aafp.org

American Academy of Head, Neck and Facial Pain
http://www.aacfp.org

American Academy of Hospice and Palliative Medicine
http://www.aahpm.org

American Academy of Neurological and Orthopedic Surgeons
http://www.aanos.org

American Academy of Neurology
http://www.aan.com

American Academy of Ophthalmology
http://www.aao.org

American Academy of Orthopedic Surgeons
http://www.aaos.org

American Academy of Otolaryngic Allergy
http://www.aaoaf.org

American Academy of Otolaryngology—Head and Neck Surgery
http://www.entnet.org

American Academy of Pain Medicine
http://www.painmed.org

American Academy of Pediatrics
http://www.aap.org

American Academy of Periodontology
http://www.perio.org

American Academy of Physical Medicine and Rehabilitation
http://www.aapmr.org

American Academy of Sleep Medicine
http://www.aasmnet.org

American Association for Respiratory Care
http://www.aarc.org

American Association of Blood Banks
http://www.aabb.org

American Association of Immunologists
http://www.aai.org

American Association of Neurological Surgeons
http://www.aans.org

American Association of Poison Control Centers
http://www.aapcc.org

American Association of Suicidology
http://www.suicidology.org

American Association on Mental Retardation
http://www.aamr.org

American Autoimmune Related Diseases Association
http://www.aarda.org

American Botanical Council
http://www.herbalgram.org

American Cancer Society
http://www.cancer.org

American Cleft Palate and Craniofacial Association
http://www.cleftpalate-craniofacial.org

American College Occupational and Environmental Medicine
http://www.acoem.org

American College of Allergy, Asthma and Immunology
http://www.allergy.mcg.edu

American College of Cardiology
http://www.acc.org

American College of Chest Physicians
http://www.chestnet.org

American College of Emergency Physicians
http://www.acep.com

American College of Endocrinology
http://www.aace.com/college

American College of Gastroenterology
http://www.acg.gi.org

American College of Medical Genetics
http://www.acmg.net

American College of Mohs Micrographic Surgery and Cutaneous Oncology
http://www.mohscollege.org

American College of Nutrition
http://www.am-coll-nutr.org

American College of Obstetrics and Gynecology
http://www.acog.org

American College of Physicians
http://www.acponline.org

American College of Preventive Medicine
http://www.acpm.org

American College of Radiology
http://www.acr.org

American College of Rheumatology
http://www.rheumatology.org

American College of Sports Medicine
http://www.acsm.org

American College of Surgeons
http://www.facs.org

American Council for Headache Education
http://www.achenet.org

American Dental Association
http://www.ada.org

American Diabetes Association
http://www.diabetes.org

American Dietetic Association
http://www.eatright.org

American Epilepsy Society
http://www.aesnet.org

American Foundation for the Blind
http://www.afb.org

American Foundation for Urologic Disease
http://www.afud.org

American Gastroenterology Association
http://www.gastro.org

American Geriatric Society
http://www.americangeriatrics.org

American Headache Society
http://www.ahsnet.org

American Heart Association
http://www.americanheart.org

American Hiking Society
http://www.americanhiking.org

American Industrial Hygiene Association
http://www.aiha.org

American Institute of Stress
http://www.stress.org

American Liver Foundation
http://www.liverfoundation.org

American Lung Association
http://www.lungusa.org

American Medical Association
http://www.ama-assn.org

American Medical Women's Association
http://www.amwa-doc.org

American Obesity Association
http://www.obesity.org

American Orthopedic Foot and Ankle Society
http://www.aofas.org

American Osteopathic Association
http://www.aoa.net

American Pain Foundation
http://www.painfoundation.org

American Pain Society
http://www.ampainsoc.org

American Parkinsons Disease Association
http://www.apdaparkinson.com

American Physical Therapy Association
http://www.apta.org

American Podiatric Medical Association
http://www.apma.org

American Psychiatric Association
http://www.psych.org

American Psychological Association
http://www.apa.org

American Psychosomatic Society
http://www.psychosomatic.org

American Social Health Association
http://www.ashastd.org

American Society for Bariatric Surgery
http://www.asbs.org

American Society for Clinical Nutrition
http://www.ascn.org

American Society for Dermatologic Surgery
http://www.asds-net.org

American Society for Nutritional Sciences
http://www.nutrition.org

American Society for Reproductive Medicine
http://www.asrm.org

American Society for Surgery of the Hand
http://www.assh.org

American Society for Therapeutic Radiology and Oncology
http://www.astro.org

American Society of Anesthesiologists
http://www.asahq.org

American Society of Cataract and Refractive Surgery
http://www.ascrs.org

American Society of Clinical Oncology
http://www.asco.org

American Society of Colon and Rectal Surgeons
http://www.fascrs.org

American Society of Cytopathology
http://www.cytopathology.org

American Society of Hematology
http://www.hematology.org

American Society of Pediatric Hematology and Oncology
http://www.aspho.org

American Society of Plastic and Reconstructive Surgeons
http://www.plasticsurgery.org

American Society of Preventive Oncology
http://www.aspo.org

American Society of Tropical Medicine and Hygiene
http://www.astmh.org

American Tinnitus Association
http://www.ata.org

American Thyroid Association
http://www.thyroid.org

American Urological Association
http://www.auanet.org

Anxiety Disorders Association of America
http://www.adaa.org

Arthritis Foundation
http://www.arthritis.org

Association for Retarded Citizens
http://www.thearc.org

Association of American Medical Colleges
http://www.aamc.org

Association Public Health Laboratories
http://www.aphl.org

Association Reproductive Health Professionals
http://www.arhp.org

Asthma and Allergy Foundation of America
http://www.aafa.org

Baylor College of Medicine
http://www.bcm.tmc.edu

Blood and Marrow Transplant Information Network
http://www.bmtinfonet.org

Brain Injury Association
http://www.biausa.org

Breast Cancer Action
http://www.bcaction.org

Breast Cancer Research
http://www.breast-cancer-research.com

Buying Medical Products Online
http://www.fda.gov/oc/buyonline

Cancer Care
http://www.cancercare.org

Celiac Disease Foundation
http://www.celiac.org

Celiac Sprue Association
http://www.csaceliacs.org

Center for Eating Disorders
http://www.eatingdisorders.org

Center for Mindfullness in Medicine, Healthcare and Society
http://www.umassmed.edu.cfm/

Center for Nutrition Policy Promotion
http://www.usda.gov/cnpp

CenterWatch Clinical Trials Listing Service
http://www.centerwatch.com

Centers for Disease Control and Prevention
http://www.cdc.gov

Centers for Disease Control and Prevention/Travel Health
http://www.cdc.gov/travel

Childbirth
http://www.childbirth.org

Children and Adults with Attention Deficit/Hyperactivity Disorder
http://www.chadd.org

Cleveland Clinic
http://www.clevelandclinic.org

ClinicalTrials.gov
http://www.clinicaltrials.gov

Contact Lens Manufacturing Association
http://www.contactlens.org

Consumer Product Safety Commission
http://www.cpsc.gov

Cornell University Center for Male Reproductive Medicine and Microsurgery
http://www.maleinfertility.org

Cornell University Center for Reproductive Medicine and Infertility
http://www.ivf.org

Crohn's and Colitis Foundation of America
http://www.ccfa.org

Cyberdiet
http://www.cyberdiet.com

CyberPsychLinks
http://www.cyberpsych.org

Cystic Fibrosis Foundation
http://www.cff.org

Diabetes Public Health Resource
http://www.cdc.gov/diabetes

Dietary Guidelines/American Heart Association
http://www.americanheart.org

Digestive Health and Nutrition Foundation
http://www.fdhn.org

Dr. Ornish Lifestyle Program
http://www.webmd.com

Drug Info Net
http://www.druginfonet.com

Duke University Health
http://www.healthydevil.studentaffairs.duke.edu

eFit (Nutricise.com)
http://www.efit.com

Emory University
http://www.medweb.emory.edu/medweb

Endocrine Society
http://www.endo-society.org

Epilepsy Foundation
http://www.epilepsyfoundation.org

Eye Surgery Education Council
http://www.lasikinstitute.org

FDA Center for Drug Evaluation and Research
http://www.fda.gov/cder

FDA Center for Food Safety and Applied Nutrition
http://www.cfsan.fda.gov

FDA Office of Women's Health
http://www.fda.gov/womens/default.htm

Fitness Center
http://www.justmove.org

Food Allergy and Anaphylaxis Network
http://www.foodallergy.org

Food and Drug Administration
http://www.fda.gov

Food and Nutrition Board/Institute of Medicine
http://www.iom.edu

Food and Nutrition Information Center
http://www.nal.usda.gov/fnic

Food Safety.Gov
http://www.foodsafety.gov

Food Standards Agency
http://www.foodstandards.gov.uk

Gambler's Anonymous International
http://www.gamblersanonymous.org

Gerontological Society of America
http://www.geron.org

George Washington Institute for Spirituality and Health
http://www.gwish.org

Glaucoma Research Foundation
http://www.glaucoma.org

Global Health and Fitness
http://www.global-fitness.com

Google
http://www.google.com

Great Outdoors Recreation Page
http://www.gorp.com

Harvard Medical School/Consumer Health
http://www.intellihealth.com

Harvard School of Dental Medicine
http://www.hsdm.med.harvard.edu

Harvard School of Public Health
http://www.hsph.harvard.edu

Health on the Net Foundation
http://www.hon.ch

Healthfinder
http://www.healthfinder.gov

Health.gov/Dietary Guidelines
http://www.health.gov/dietaryguidelines

Healthy People 2010
http://www.healthypeople.gov

Hepatitis Foundation International
http://www.hepfi.org

Hospice Net
http://www.hospicenet.org

Huffington Center on Aging/Baylor College of Medicine
http://www.hcoa.org

Human Cloning Foundation
http://www.humancloning.org

Institute of Medicine/Health Information
http://www.iom.edu

Interactive Healthy Eating Index
http://www.usda.gov/cnpp

International Federation of Multiple Sclerosis Societies
http://www.msif.org/en/

International Food and Information Council
http://www.ific.org

International Foundation for Functional Gastrointestinal Disorders
http://www.iffgd.org

International Hyperhydrosis Society
http://www.sweathelp.org

International Society for Heart and Lung Transplantation
http://www.ishlt.org

International Society of Refractive Surgery
http://www.isrs.org

Internet Hospital Directory
http://www.bowyer.org.uk/hospital.htm

Internet Medical School Directory
http://www.bowyer.org/uk/med_sch.htm

Interstitial Cystitis Association
http://www.ichelp.org

Iron Disorders Institute
http://www.irondisorders.org

Johns Hopkins University Medical Center
http://www.hopkinsmedicine.org

Just Move.org
http://www.justmove.org

Juvenile Diabetes Research Foundation
http://www.jdrf.org

Karolinska Institute
http://www.mic.ki.se

Kid's Health
http://www.kidshealth.org

Komen Breast Cancer Foundation
http://www.komen.org

Lab Tests Online
http://www.labtestsonline.net

Learning Disabilities Association of America
http://www.ldantl.org

Leukemia and Lymphoma Society
http://www.leukemia.org

Lighthouse International
http://www.lighthouse.org

Lupus Foundation of American
http://www.lupus.org

Mayo Clinic
http://www.mayoclinic.com

Med Help International
http://www.medhelp.org

Medical College of Wisconsin/Healthlink
http://www.mcw.edu

Medicare
http://www.medicare.gov

Medline
http://medline.cos.com

Medlineplus
http://www.medlineplus.gov

Mental Health Net
http://www.mentalhelp.net

Mind/Body Medical Institute
http://www.mbmi.org

Movement Disorder Society
http://www.wemove.org

Muscular Dystrophy Association
http://www.mdausa.org

Myositis Association of America
http://www.myositis.org

National Academy for Child Development
http://www.nacd.org

National Academy of Science
http://www.nas.edu

National Acupuncture and Oriental Medicine Alliance
http://www.acuall.org

National Adrenal Diseases Foundation
http://www.medhelp.org/nadf/

National Alliance for the Mentally Ill
http://www.nami.org

National Association for Continence
http://www.nafc.org

National Association for Down Syndrome
http://www.nads.org

National Association for Home Care
http://www.nahc.org

National Association of Anorexia and Related Disorders
http://www.anad.org

National Cancer Institute
http://www.cancer.gov

National Center for Chronic Disease Prevention and Health Promotion
http://www.cdc.gov/nccdphp/dnpa

National Center for Complimentary and Alternative Medicine
http://www.nccam.nih.gov

National Center for Elder Abuse
http://www.elderabusecenter.org

National Center for Injury Prevention and Control
http://www.cdc.gov/ncipc

National Center for Posttraumatic Stress Disorder
http://www.ncptsd.org

National Center on Sleep Disorders Research
http://www.nhlbi.nih.gov/about/ncsdr/index.htm

National Chronic Fatigue and Fibromyalgia Association
http://www.cfidsfoundation.org

National Coalition for Cancer Survivorship
http://www.canceradvocacy.org

National Council on Alcoholism and Drug Dependence
http://www.ncadd.net

National Council on Problem Gambling
http://www.ncpgambling.org

National Down Syndrome Society
http://www.ndss.org

National Eye Institute
http://www.nei.nih.gov

National Family Caregivers Association
http://www.nfcacares.org

National Foundation for Infectious Diseases
http://www.nfid.org

National Guideline Clearinghouse
http://www.guideline.gov

National Headache Foundation
http://www.headaches.org

National Heart, Lung and Blood Institute
http://www.nhlbi.nih.gov

National Hospice and Palliative Care Organization
http://www.hospiceinfo.org

National Human Genome Research Institute
http://www.nhgri.nih.gov

National Institute for Occupational Safety and Health
http://www.cdc.gov/niosh

National Institute of Allergy and Infectious Disease
http://www.niaid.nih.gov

National Institute of Arthritis and Musculoskeletal and Skin Diseases
http://www.niams.nih.gov

National Institute of Child Health and Human Development
http://www.nichd.nih.gov

National Institute of Dental and Craniofacial Research
http://www.nidcr.nih.gov

National Institute of Diabetes and Digestive and Kidney Diseases
http://www.niddk.nih.gov

National Institute of Environmental Health Sciences
http://www.niehs.nih.gov

National Institute of Mental Health
http://www.nimh.nih.gov

National Institute of Neurological Disorders and Stroke
http://www.ninds.nih.gov

National Institute on Aging
http://www.nia.nih.gov

National Institute on Alcohol Abuse and Alcoholism
http://www.niaaa.nih.gov

National Institute on Deafness and Other Communication Disorders
http://www.nidcd.nih.gov

National Institute on Drug Abuse
http://www.nida.nih.gov

National Institutes of Health/Health Information
http://www.health.nih.gov

National Kidney Foundation
http://www.kidney.org

National Library of Medicine
http://www.nlm.nih.gov

National Lymphedema Network
http://www.lymphnet.org

National Mental Health Association
http://www.nmha.org

National Multiple Sclerosis Society
http://www.nmss.org

National Osteoporosis Foundation
http://www.nof.org

National Ovarian Cancer Coalition
http://www.ovarian.org

National Parkinson Foundation
http://www.parkinson.org

National Psoriasis Foundation
http://www.psoriasis.org

National Right to Life
http://www.nrlc.org/abortion

National Senior Citizens Law Center
http://www.nsclc.org

National Sleep Foundation
http://www.sleepfoundation.org

National Stroke Association
http://www.stroke.org

National Spasmodic Torticollis Association
http://www.torticollis.org

National Wellness Institute
http://www.nationalwellness.org

National Women's Health Information Center
http://www.4women.org

National Women's Health Resource Center
http://www.healthywomen.org

Net Wellness
http://www.netwellness.org

New York Online Access to Health
http://www.noah-health.org

North American Menopause Society
http://www.menopause.org

Nutrition.Gov
http://www.nutrition.gov

Occupational Safety and Health Administration
http://www.osha.gov

Office of Dietary Supplements
http://ods.od.info.nih.gov

Office of Disease Prevention and Health Promotion
http://www.od.nih.gov

Office of Rare Diseases/National Institutes of Health
http://www.rarediseases.info.nih.gov/ord

Oncology Nursing Society
http://www.ons.org

Outdoors.org
http://www.outdoors.org

Ovarian Cancer National Alliance
http://www.ovariancancer.org

Paget's Disease Foundation
http://www.paget.org

Parkinson Disease Foundation
http://www.pdf.org

Patient Advocate Foundation
http://www.patientadvocate.org

Planned Parenthood Federation of America
http://www.ppfa.org

Posttraumatic Stress Disorder Alliance
http://www.ptsdalliance.org

President's Council on Physical Fitness and Sports
http://www.fitness.gov

Prevent Blindness America
http://www.preventblindness.org

Prostateinfo.com
http://www.prostateinfo.com

PubMed
http://www.ncbi.nlm.nih.gov/pubmed

Rational Recovery Systems
http://www.rational.org

Recreation.gov
http://www.recreation.gov

Rx List/The Internet Drug Index
http://www.rxlist.com

Scleroderma Foundation
http://www.scleroderma.org

Shape Up America
http://www.shapeup.org

Shoreland's Travel Health Online
http://www.tripprep.com

Society for Adolescent Medicine
http://www.adolescenthealth.org

Society of American Gastrointestinal Endoscopic Surgeons
http://www.sages.org

Society of Critical Care Medicine
http://www.sccm.org

Society of General Internal Medicine
http://www.sgim.org

Society of Interventional Radiology
http://www.sirweb.org

Society of Nuclear Medicine
http://www.snm.org

Society of Thoracic Surgeons
http://www.sts.org

Spina Bifida Association
http://www.sbaa.org

Spine Health
http://www.spine-health.com

Stem Cell Research Foundation
http://www.stemcellresearchfoundation.org

Surgeon General's Office
http://www.surgeongeneral.gov/sgoffice.htm

Take Off Pounds Sensibly
http://www.tops.org

Thyroid Foundation of America
http://www.tsh.org

Thyroid Society
http://www.the-thyroid-society.org

Trichotillomania Learning Center
http://www.trich.org

Tufts Nutritional Navigator
http://navigator.tufts.edu

UCLA Medical Center
http://www.healthcare.ucla.edu

United Cerebral Palsy Association
http://www.ucpa.org

University of Pennsylvania Cancer Center/Oncolink
http://www.oncolink.upenn.edu

University of Virginia Healthsystem
http://www.healthsystem.virginia.edu

US Administration on Aging
http://www.aoa.dhhs.gov

US Department of Health and Human Services
http://www.os.dhhs.gov

USDA Center for Nutrition Policy Promotion
http://www.usda.gov/cnpp

USDA Food and Nutrition Information Center
http://www.nal.usda.gov/fnic

USDA Nutrient Data Laboratory
http://www.nal.usda.gov/fnic/foodcomp

USDA Phytonutrient Laboratory
http://www.barc.usda.gov/bhnrc/pl

Vegetarian Resource Group
http://www.vrg.org

Vanderbilt University Medical Center
http://www.mc.vanderbilt.edu

Veterans Affairs Health
http://www1.va.gov/health_benefits

WebMd
http://www.webmd.com

Wellness Community
http://www.wellness-community.org

Women's Health Matters Network
http://www.womenshealthmatters.ca

World Health Organization
http://www.who.int

Your Surgery.com
http://www.yoursurgery.com

About the Author

Eugene A. De Felice, M.D., is an internationally recognized author, educator, and retired Distinguished Clinical Professor of Medicine (Robert Wood Johnson Medical School) who is listed in the prestigious Marquis': Who's Who in Medicine and Healthcare, Who's Who in America, and Who's Who in the World. He is the author of numerous medical/scientific articles published in professional journals and 10 key books on medicine, nutrition and health, and Web Health Resources including:

1. Web Health Information Resources, Second Edition, iUniverse Inc., 2004
2. Nutrition and Health, iUniverse Inc, 2003
3. Overweight, Obesity and Health, iUniverse Inc, 2002.
4. Breast Cancer, iUniverse Inc, 2002
5. Web Health Information Resource Guide, iUniverse Inc, 2001
6. Angiotensin Converting Enzyme Inhibitors, Alan R. Liss, 1987
7. Pharmaeological Treatment of Cardiovascular Disease, Elsevier, 1986
8. Beta Blockers in the Treatment of Cardiovascular Disease, Raven Press, 1984
9. Health and Obesity, Raven Press, 1983
10. Protaglandins, Platelets, Lipids: New Developments in Atherosclerosis, Elsevier, 1981

0-595-32628-5